DOCTOR GOLDMAN'S
GUIDE
(TO)
EFFECTIVE
PATIENT
COMMUNICATION

Explanations of the Most Common
Medical Conditions in Layperson's Terms
And Helpful Provider-Patient Interactions

KISSINGER GOLDMAN, DO, MBA

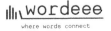

where words connect

DOCTOR GOLDMAN'S
GUIDE
(TO)
EFFECTIVE
PATIENT
COMMUNICATION

Explanations of the Most Common
Medical Conditions in Layperson's Terms
And Helpful Provider-Patient Interactions

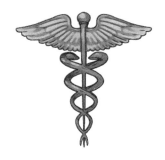

Doctor Goldman's Guide to Effective Patient Communication
Explanations of the Most Common Medical Conditions in Layperson's
Terms And Helpful Provider-Patient Interactions

First edition
ISBN: (Paperback) 978-1-959811-12-1
ISBN: (e-book) 978-1-959811-13-8
Library of Congress Control Number: 2023908119

Illustrations: Zac Crawford
Cover Design: Okomota
Cover Photo: Joshua Prezant
Interior Design: Amit Dey

Website: www.wordeee.com
Twitter: wordeeeupdates
Facebook: facebook.com/wordeee/
e-mail: contact@wordeee.com

Published by Wordeee in the United States, Beacon, New York, 2023

Printed in the USA

Dr. Goldman's training website: Howtopatient.com

LEGAL DISCLAIMER:

The following legal disclaimer governs the use of *Doctor Goldman's Guide to Effective Patient Communication: Explanations of the Most Common Medical Conditions in Layperson's Terms and Helpful Provider-Patient Interactions* ("Manual"). By accessing and utilizing this Manual, you acknowledge and agree to the terms outlined below:

1. No Legal Advice: The information contained in this Manual is provided for educational and informational purposes only. It is not intended as legal advice or to create an attorney-client relationship. The Manual does not substitute for professional legal advice, and you should consult with a qualified legal professional regarding your specific circumstances or concerns.

2. Accuracy and Completeness: While Dr. Kissinger Goldman strives to ensure the accuracy and completeness of the information provided in the Manual, he makes no representations or warranties of any kind, express or implied, about the accuracy, reliability, or suitability of the content. You acknowledge that any reliance you place on the information in this Manual is at your own risk.

3. Personal Responsibility: The content provided in this Manual is designed to enhance patient experience training and improve healthcare services. However, the implementation and application of these guidelines are your responsibility. Dr Kissinger Goldman shall not be held liable for any direct, indirect, incidental, consequential, or punitive damages arising out of the use of this Manual.

4. Intellectual Property: The Manual and all related materials, including but not limited to text, graphics, logos, and images, are protected by intellectual property laws and are the sole property of Dr. Kissinger Goldman. Unauthorized reproduction, distribution, or use of any part of this Manual is strictly prohibited.

5. External Links: This Manual may contain links to external websites or resources maintained by third parties. These links are provided for convenience and do not signify endorsement or responsibility for the content, accuracy, or availability of these external resources. Dr. Kissinger Goldman shall not be held liable for any damages or loss arising from the use of such external links.

6. Modifications: Dr. Kissinger Goldman reserves the right to modify, update, or discontinue the content of this Manual at any time without prior notice. We encourage users to regularly review the Manual to ensure compliance with the most recent version.

7. Applicable Law: This Manual and its legal disclaimer shall be governed by and construed in accordance with the laws of Florida. Any disputes arising out of or in connection with this Manual shall be subject to the exclusive jurisdiction of the courts in Florida.

By using this Manual, you acknowledge that you have read, understood, and agreed to the terms and conditions of this legal disclaimer. If you do not agree with any part of this disclaimer, please refrain from using the manual.

TESTIMONIALS

"I am the CEO of Memorial Hospital West. I reviewed Dr. Goldman's book and, wow, I really enjoyed the experience. The book teaches effective stylistic approaches that can improve patient-physician relationships and foster enhanced communication. It also offers vital strategies that can be used to improve our interactions with our clients. Goldman offers deep insights that will help us connect with our patients and families and improve their care experience journey."

Everyone involved in patient care will benefit from the real-life situations and answers presented here.

—Vedner Guerrier
Chief Executive Officer
Memorial Hospital West

As a Nurse Practitioner and also a Chief Executive Officer, I understand on multiple levels the importance of the patient's experience within a health care institution. I strongly believe that this manuscript can be (and should be) utilized to educate physicians, allied staff, and employees about how to improve the patient's experience. This book is truly an invaluable tool!

—Grisel Fernandez-Bravo, APRN, MBA, DNP
Chief Executive Officer
MHS Staffing Resources

During our medical training we learn how to perform histories and physicals, develop differential diagnoses, order, and interpret tests, and arrive at the best treatment plans for our patients. What we don't learn is how to effectively communicate with those patients. Doctor Goldman's Guide is a book that all medical professionals need to read in order to learn how to communicate in a clear, concise manner, and, most importantly, in a way that patients will understand!

—Ryan Voccia
Emergency Medicine Physician Assistant

During my training I heard many doctors talk about to a something called "The Art of Medicine"—the way in which medical professionals effectively interact with their clients. But in all that time I never came across a book or training manual on the subject. The 'Art' was something that I learned through trial and error, and through the stories and anecdotes of my professors. Goldman's manuscript to successfully communicate and interact with their patients and colleagues. This is what medicine is all about: knowledge, empathy, and the ability to make a difference. I wish I had read this manuscript in medical school and in residency. I highly recommend it, and very much hope there will be another volume.

—Tahnie Danastor, MD, FACOG

As a current medical student, I believe 'The Goldman Guide' provides an invaluable resource for those transitioning into their clinical rotations. Dr. Goldman has always been a role model and fierce advocate for hospital staff camaraderie, patient care, and most importantly, patient communication. With this guide, we can endeavor to improve the healthcare experience for everyone involved.

—Jonathan Muñoz,
Medical Student

Simple, yet powerful! Dr. Goldman has developed the secret sauce that optimizes the provider-patient relationship and improves the quality of patient care, patient outcomes, and the overall patient experience. Patients will rave about the providers who consistently apply these practices.

The healthcare industry continues to experience rapid changes, and institutions that wish to stay relevant must find simple and effective ways to 'meet patients where they are' as they endeavor to deliver great care. This book is a highly effective tool that can help providers connect with their patients in a more meaningful ways, in order to improve outcomes.

This manuscript is a much-needed resource for new medical providers who are being on-boarded into an ever-changing medical environment that promotes the notion that effective provider/patient interactions overwhelmingly lead to better medical results.

—Julie Staub
Executive Vice President &
Chief Human Resources Officer
Jackson Health System

Dr. Goldman's Treatise is a "Must Read" for any physician, nurse, or support staff member. Numerous medical negligence claims get filed because patients and family members are excluded from the dialogue: are not told of diagnostic test results, consequential lab findings or discharge instructions. Many families seek legal assistance, even when the best of care may have been provided, because they "don't really know what happened."

—David B. Mishael, Esquire
Malpractice Attorney

Dr Goldman's Guide to Effective Patient Communication addresses a major gap in medical education by offering a concise and practical approach to provider-patient interactions. It provides effective conversation tools which led to a better healthcare experience for all involved. This book should be incorporated into any curriculum that trains providers to care for patients."

—Michael T Dalley, DO FAAEM
Program Director Emergency Medicine Residency
Mount Sinai Medical Center Miami Beach
Clinical Associate Professor, Department of Emergency
Medicine Herbert Wertheim College of Medicine,
Florida International University Clinical Assistant Professor,
Department of Emergency Medicine
Dr. Kiran C. Patel College of Osteopathic Medicine,
NOVA Southeastern University

The Goldman Doctor-Patient Guide To Effective Communication succeeds in the reorientation of the physician and other caregivers from a purely diagnostic orientation to a communication mindset. This guide recognizes that the patient is far more than a number, in fact there's commonly a person and an entire family to consider when providing care in a hospital setting. This guide will help caregivers to focus on empathy, effective communication and better outcomes.

—Jose Basulto, MBA, CPA
Commissioner, Memorial Healthcare System
Hollywood, Florida

In this guide, Dr. Goldman provides an insightful and interesting read related to patient communication and satisfaction. Each section provides a concise perspective with solid recommendations on how to handle some of the most challenging aspects related to communication in the care of a patient.

—Robert T. Hasty, DO, FACOI, FACP
Dean & Chief Academic Officer,
Orlando College of Osteopathic Medicine - OCOM

TABLE OF CONTENTS

Dedication xix

Author's Note xxi

**SECTION I: The Benefits of Effective
Communication** 1

The Impact of Effective Communication On Patients 3

The Impact of Effective Communication On Providers . . 4

The Impact Of Effective Communication On Healthcare
Systems 5

Quiz: The Benefits of Effective Communication . . . 7

Healthcare Workers' Comments On The Impact Of
Effective Communications 9

Complaints 15

Who Complains About Patient Care? 19

Improve The Patient Experience .23

Entering The Patient's Room 26

The Physical Examination 30

The Plan of Care 32

Results and Disposition 34

The Discharge Process 37

Special Cases 39

Other Factors that Impact The Patient. 42

Quiz: How Can a Patient Be Satisfied? 45

Managing Expectations 53

Quiz: Managing Expectations 56

SECTION II: This, That, and The Other. 58

After The Patient Goes Home. 60

Provider Callback: Who Do I Call Back? When?
What Should I Expect? 61

Quiz: After the Patient Goes Home. 64

WHY? 66

Quiz: Why? 70

CAVEATS. 72

Quiz: Caveats 82

Moral Dilemma. 86

Quiz: Moral Dilemma 89

Sexual and Gender Identification 90

Quiz: Sexual and Gender Identification 92

Eight Hours 94

Quiz: Eight Hours 96

SECTION III: Special Attention **97**

The Pediatric Experience 99

    Quiz: The Pediatric Experience 101

I Want a Medical Test! 102

    Quiz: Medical Tests 104

Improving The Ancillary Staff's Experience 105

    Quiz: Improving The Ancillary Staff's Experience 107

Engaging The Nursing Staff 108

    Quiz: Engaging the Nursing Staff 110

Lessons From the Pandemic 111

Covid-19 Remote Family Communication Tips. 115

    Quiz: Lessons from the Pandemic. 117

Relationships in Healthcare. 119

    Quiz: Relationships in Healthcare. 123

The Other Side. 124

    Quiz: The Other Side. 125

SECTION IV: Patient Speak. 126

Trauma: What Your Patients Should Know 128

Head, Ears, Eyes, Nose, Throat 135

Neurological. 135

Psychological 137

Cardiovascular. 137

Pulmonary 139

Gastrointestinal 142

Endocrine. 146

Urological. 147

Urogenital. 149

Musculoskeletal. 149

Skin 151

Oncological 152

Hematological 153

Infectious Disease 153

Quiz: Patient Speak. 155

SECTION V: Case Studies **164**

Case 1 166

Lessons Learned 167

Case 2 168

Case 3 168

Case 4 169

Case 6 170

Case 7 171

Case 8 171

Case 9 173

Case 10 173

Case 11 174

Conclusion 176

Acknowledgements 179

DEDICATION

This book is dedicated to my mom, Antonia Bernard. Leaving Haiti to support your newly fatherless children, going to school as an adult, working multiple jobs, cooking, raising four kids are only some of the accomplishments that make you my hero. Thank you for your patience. Thank you for your unconditional love. Thank you for helping me become the man I am today.

AUTHOR'S NOTE

Think about the last time someone you know was in the hospital or visited a doctor. If you are in the healthcare profession, chances are your friend called you right afterwards to help them make sense of what their doctor had just told them. When patients have a friend or family member in the medical field, they will often automatically make them their default expert on all things medical. But the bigger question is, "Why would a patient have to call their friend or family member for a clearer explanation of their medical condition that they just consulted the doctor about?" The answer lies in the type of communication that occurs between the healthcare provider and the patient.

I have been a Patient Experience Improvement Consultant for over a decade. In that time, I have witnessed countless avoidable situations and reviewed numerous records of patients with negative outcomes who became dissatisfied patients. The two most common reasons for these negative outcomes are:

1. Patients failing to understand their diagnosis and/or their plan of care
2. The healthcare providers' disposition

To help address these issues at the medical facility where I am on staff, I found myself teaching colleagues things that they should have learned at some point in their training but didn't. Firstly, how to translate academic training practices and medical jargon into simple terms that can be understood by a layperson. Secondly, how to deliver essential information to patients in a manner that fosters trust and compliance. I have modeled this behavior early on and, as a result I was asked to become the Director of Patient Experience at my healthcare system. My experiences in this role have reinforced how critical these two elements are in reducing negative patient experiences.

My own medical training was a mixed bag when it came to connecting with patients. I was mentored by several great clinical teachers, some of whom had impeccable bedside manners, many of which I still emulate today. Unfortunately, I also experienced mentorship by other clinicians who, while excellent, exhibited behaviors towards their patients and their families that were less than desirable.

Most of my teachers did a great job in teaching me the technical aspects of medicine, including how to effectively diagnose and treat heart attacks, strokes, pneumonia, and so much more. However, what some teachers failed to convey was that while the right diagnosis is important, the manner in which physicians explain the diagnosis and the plan of care to our patients and their loved ones, is equally as important. In today's health care system, the old ways of ' treat them and street them' must be replaced with genuine connection and effective communication between the healthcare providers and their patients. You will find myriad reasons for this shift in healthcare emphasis outlined in this book.

Doctor Goldman's Guide to Effective Patient Communication has information I wish I had known when I started my clinical rotations so many years ago. The data was collected from hundreds of thousands of patient comments about their healthcare providers, and from healthcare systems all around the country. In addition to reviewing all the data, I have spoken to a vast number of patients, healthcare providers and hospital administrators on the topic. This book directs you to proven patient engagement techniques, all gleaned from synthesizing, and analyzing the compiled data on the subject. These techniques have been successfully put into practice at a number of healthcare centers, including my own.

Additionally, the book contains a compilation of patient-focused explanations for the most common medical conditions. I find it incredible that even today, I still hear residents telling patients that they have "diverticulitis" without defining exactly what that medical condition is. Explaining a diagnosis to a patient in clear and concise language builds trust and motivates the patient to comply with the important medical instructions given. When patients understand their diagnosis and treatment plan, they will take ownership of their care. Taking ownership of one's care is a key predictor of better healthcare outcomes.

I urge you to use the material contained in the following pages. The information will help to improve your communication with patients and families and decrease the number of patient complaints attributed to you or to your institution. Adapt the suggested communication techniques to your style, including utilizing layman definitions of medical conditions to inform your word choices when speaking to patients. I believe this will help your communication to be clear, concise and most of all, understood. Using this manual *will* ultimately help you to improve patient care, an outcome we all desire as health professionals. Successful patient engagement is rooted in effective communication, and that is why I am positive that you will find this information helpful for you and for your patients.

Kissinger Goldman DO, MBA

June 2023

www.kissingergoldman.com

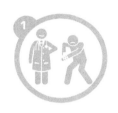

THE BENEFITS OF EFFECTIVE COMMUNICATION

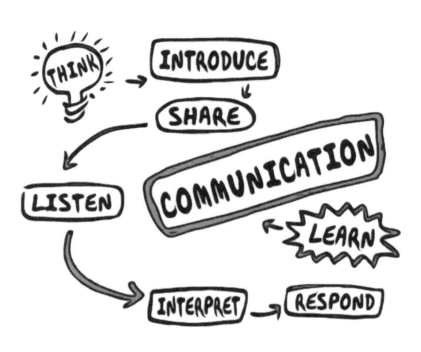

The Impact of Effective Communication On Patients

The data points clearly to the fact that patients who have effective interactions with their healthcare providers are more cooperative, more likely to follow up, and more likely to cease harmful habits impacting their health, such as smoking. They are also less likely to suffer from the acute medical emergencies that require the need for urgent care in the emergency room. Because of *your* effective communication skills, patients will now be able to understand and take charge of their disease processes in a helpful way while under your care and beyond. Some of them may even go one step further and become healthcare advocates for their family and friends.

Effective doctor/patient interactions open the lines of communication, which engender trust and lead to better care. Even after being discharged, patients and their family members are more willing to contact the healthcare provider they have formed a relationship with, if new symptoms arise or if they have specific questions. They are not so inclined to do the same with providers with whom no meaningful relationship exists. Creating a safe place for dialogue empowers patients and their families to proactively take charge of their health.

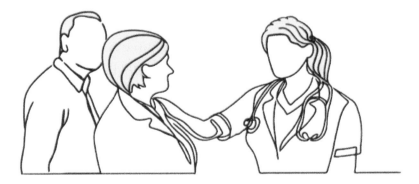

The Impact of Effective Communication On Providers

When I've had a positive interaction with a patient, I feel a mixture of satisfaction and a sense of 'mission accomplished.' This feeling is particularly enhanced when the patient or their family expresses appreciation for their care (however big or small). These 'appreciative' interactions benefit me in several ways. They:

- Give me a physical jolt, almost as if I drank a strong cup of Cuban coffee. Appreciation is the epinephrine my cells need to give me the energy to see more patients, however tired I am.

- Remind me why I went into medicine in the first place. I remember being told by one of my attending physicians during my residency that medicine is a "thankless job." It has been my experience that this belief is not true when the provider has strong patient communication skills.

- Can stoke my inner fire and keep me going when I would otherwise falter. The fact is that negative interactions between the patient and the provider can douse the fire that inspired us to go to medical school in the first place. This is a mindset to be avoided at all costs.

- Bolster my enthusiasm, and enthusiasm is contagious. When I am on shift and I'm excited and positive, I notice a lot more smiles around me - not only among physicians but also with the nurses, x-ray techs, ultrasonographers, custodians, and patients. The morale and job satisfaction of the entire team can be impacted by the disposition of a single provider.

- Provide me with an anchor when I am having a bad shift. There are difficult days for me in the ER, marked by dangerously high patient volume, acutely sick patients, slow lab results, broken CT scan machines, and so much more. Boosted by each positive interaction, I can get through these days, and I can power through temporary setbacks.

The Impact Of Effective Communication On Healthcare Systems

To our delight, patients have stated that they bypass a number of healthcare establishments just to come to our facilities. We have patients who will wait for hours to be seen by one of our care team staff, rather than go to another healthcare center. This validates our commitment to enhancing effective provider/patient communication, as well as, our success in doing so. It is such an uplifting feeling when patients make statements like, "It's because of the way you guys care about me."

After combing through thousands of patients' comments, and after making countless post-visit calls to patients to understand why, the data is unmistakable; the 'care' our patients are referring to is the manner in which our providers communicate with them. The 'care' is directly linked to our effective and quality communication strategies, the bedrock of our facility. Enhanced patient interaction training is a requirement for all providers who work at my healthcare center. This training is rooted in the work culture of the facility, and it has inspired our team to always aim to surpass patient expectations.

Healthcare providers can play a critical role in determining whether patients understand, accept, and follow through on our medical advice. Patients are more likely to accept and follow through on our recommendations if they sense the advice given is coming from a caring provider rather than from just another medical professional whose expertise is imparted to them in a dispassionate way. When a provider has been trained to use vocal tone, eye contact, body language, and body positioning to project a genuine sense of caring, patients are more likely to trust, appreciate and accept their treatment plans, and have positive health outcomes.

Quiz: The Benefits of Effective Communication

1. Which of the following are the benefits of effective patient/provider communication?

    A. Patients are more likely to cease a harmful habit such as smoking.

    B. Patients are less likely to suffer from acute medical emergencies.

    C. Patients can understand and take charge of their disease processes.

    D. All of the above.

    Answer: D

2. Effective communication between a provider and a patient can result in the patient becoming a healthcare advocate for their family and friends.

    A. True

    B. False

    Answer: A

3. Effective provider/patient interactions will likely create a safe space for e patients to initiate communication with their providers after being discharged, if new symptoms arise.

   A. True

   B. False

   Answer: A

4. Effective communication and interaction between providers and patients will most likely _____ patients to proactively participate in their health care journey.

   A. Discourage

   B. Empower

   C. Prevent

   D. Reject

   Answer: B

5. Positive interactions between staff and patients tend to:

   A. Motivate and engage healthcare staff.

   B. Provide job satisfaction to healthcare staff.

   C. Boost morale among the healthcare staff.

   D. All of the above.

   Answer: D

Healthcare Workers' Comments On The Impact Of Effective Communications

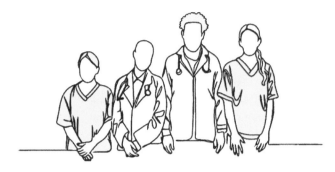

The following are actual responses from members of the Memorial Hospital West team to questions asked about the impact and benefits of a positive attitude and effective communication delivered to patients with empathy. Respondents included:

- Michael Rodriguez., ER Paramedic, 9 years in current position

- Vedner Guerrier., CEO, Memorial Hospital West, 6 months in current position; 21 years at Memorial Healthcare System

- LaShonda Rogers, Unit Coordinator: 15 years

- Gloria Almodóvar, Director of Emergency Services, 3 years

- Deedra Satahoo, ER Nurse, 15 years in current position

What impact (if any) have you seen on the staff when providers have a positive attitude?

- A positive provider attitude impacts the staff, and that positivity is infectious. It helps boost morale and keeps the stress level down.

- The staff is more engaged, and the physician has a more aligned team supporting their needs and that of their patients.

- Positivity is contagious! Providers are seen as leaders amongst our staff, and the staff look up to them; so, their behavior is very impactful.

- The impact I have seen on the staff when providers have a positive attitude is that the atmosphere is less tense. There is room for open communication on all matters concerning the patient. Staff members therefore feel more confident when approaching the provider with any questions or concerns. ultimately resulting in a better outcome for the patient.

How has the positive attitude of a provider professionally or personally impacted you as a team member?

- Personally, I admire it when a provider has a positive personality regardless of how stressful a situation can be. As a former soldier, we were taught to have "military bearing" which is the ability to stay calm, focused, and keep your emotions out of the equation under any circumstance. Providers with that ability have earned my respect

- Having a physician who focuses on being positive allows me to work collaboratively with them. Our collective skills can be used to resolve the challenges before us in a collegial manner. Professionally, I seek out these types of physicians for their feedback and guidance

- Positive teamwork is the major impact I have witnessed with the staff when the providers display a positive attitude. Everyone works together, everyone listens to each other, all of which increase motivation promotes better decision making, and enables the team to achieve the most ideal outcome for the patient

- Professionally, the positive attitude of a provider has impacted me in so many ways. It motivates me to be the best that I can be in my daily job duties. It keeps me from making mistakes that can jeopardize my job performance. Also, it reduces the stressful work environment

- Personally, a positive provider attitude helps me feel respected as a team member. As an individual I have opened up to positive-attitude providers, sometimes discussing my personal future endeavors with them. Their encouraging words have been a major encouraging factor in helping me achieve my goals

- Having positive collaborations with other physicians and/or physician leaders is imperative to my success. It makes me feel like we're on the same team and that we are moving in the same direction with common goals. It's powerful!

- The positive attitude of a provider professionally impacts me because I feel like a valued member of the care team. The provider's positivity and excitement fosters a culture of great patient care. It allows for different treatment strategies to be discussed with the inclusion of the patient and family, resulting in greater improvements in outcome. These improvements always lead to greater patient satisfaction scores. The patients understand that everyone caring for them is actually working as a team, and that their best interests are at the heart of our team. Staff morale improves in proportion to good satisfaction scores and positive feedback from patients. As a result, the staff members look forward to coming to work each day, they are more likely to treat each other like family. This is why our staff retention numbers are so high.

How does the patient interaction with the lead provider impact your ability to perform your duties?

- It makes my job a lot easier when the patient is well informed.

- Patients respond to effective provider communication because they are shown respect, supported, and treated with dignity. The overall patient experience is much improved when physicians make listening a priority.

- As a hospital executive, I can say without any doubt that effective physician-led communication makes my job easier. Patients are less likely to complain about care providers when the services they receive are delivered with empathy and mindfulness.

- Working as a Health Unit Coordinator has helped me appreciate just how much direct contact and good verbal communication strategies are needed in order to deliver effective patient care. These communications include direct contact with other providers such as informing them, "I'm going to a patient's room to get information regarding their primary care physician that I then need to deliver to the ER physician."

- Effective communication that uses clear and concise language is essential if you wish to avoid duplication of processes and circumvent misunderstandings. It is a major time saver!

What is the Impact of Effective Communication on Patient Care?

- I can focus on my duties, rather than spend my time revisiting explanations about treatment plans, diagnostic results, and/or prognoses.

- The patient experience is better. When physicians engage effectively with patients, the patient has the impression that they received quality care. Good physician engagement goes a long way. Patients embrace provider-led communication because they are shown respect, support, and treated with dignity. Physicians do a better job listening, which improves the patient's experience.

- Open communication has a major impact on the overall patient experience. One example of open communication is eye to eye contact, which is a strategy to show the patient that you are very focused on their concerns. As the patient-physician relationship develops, patients are more inclined to trust their provider, and to become more involved in their own health care journey, which is always a positive outcome. Open communication triggers a space in which patients are more likely to share information that might have remained hidden during a formal or more uncomfortable interaction. That information they share might very well impact their diagnosis, and possibly help to determine the right treatment plan for them.

- True Patient Satisfaction! Patients come to the ER (emergency room) to see a provider for health care. In the process they will be given the provider's opinion about their health issues. Sometimes that opinion is all that matters to a patient, and the words spoken may become words that will never be forgotten.

- Positive communication with patients will often translate into a smooth, effective, and efficient delivery of healthcare, and a better chance of a positive outcome.

How does Effective Communication from the Provider impact Staff Morale?

- Effective communication can transform a mediocre medical staff team into an efficient, well-tuned machine, able to apportion time in advantageous ways for the patients. One example of this occurs when the staff team uses their time to care for the patient, rather than using it to revisit the diagnosis and treatment plan that has already been explained to the patient.

- When patients are more content, I find that my work environment feels lighter, and the workload is easier to navigate. I think everyone feels that way. This leads to a staff workday that is manageable for everyone, and more enjoyable.

- In an effective communication space, employees are able to share ideas, discuss different topics, bring up concerns with the providers, and work with the physicians to determine what is best for the patient's care. It is a space in which different skill sets and experiences collaborate to make valuable contributions, thereby improving the rapport and respect that exists between the staff and the physicians.

- Providers are seen as professional leaders, and consequently looked up to in the workplace. They can create the ideal workplace environment because the staff will model the emotions, thoughts, attitudes, and behavior that they see in the provider.

COMPLAINTS

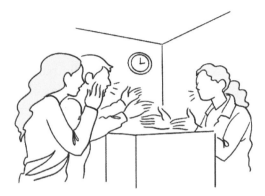

Let's talk about Patient Satisfaction. Part of my job as a Patient Experience Consultant over the past decade involves reviewing patient complaints. I have had thousands of one-on-one conversations with angry patients, and I can confidently state that patient satisfaction is not tied to giving a patient whatever they want. Nor is it about simply giving the patient pain medicine, although this might be necessary in some cases. I have found that patients who get exactly what they want, even if it is prescribed pain medication to alleviate discomfort, still overwhelmingly have complaints about the care they received. These two elements are not enough.

So, What Is Patient Satisfaction?

Patients are satisfied with their care when they have a healthcare provider who addresses their expectations, invites their participation, and invests in their comprehension. Patients are satisfied when these three elements are incorporated into their care, and when they are delivered with empathy.

Addressing Expectations

Patients walk into our healthcare centers with certain expectations. Some are upfront with their concerns. They might say, "I want to make sure I don't have brain cancer." Many come in with nonspecific complaints: "I have belly pain." Quite apart from their symptoms, the patient might be wrestling with mental or emotional stress associated with the fear of receiving bad medical news. Our job is to assess exactly what their expectations are and address them. We have patients who come in expecting to have ALL their concerns addressed in one way or another. Sometimes we may simply need to ask our patients, "What is it that you are concerned about today?"

Inviting Participation

Patients want to participate in their own care. From a clinical standpoint we encourage this because there is clear evidence that patients who are actively involved in their care have better outcomes. Patients, unless they tell us otherwise, often want their friends and families to be a part of their care team as well. Provide an opportunity during the medical interview for friends and family to contribute information that they feel the patient failed to mention. When the patient leaves our facility, their family members and their friends can serve as healthcare extenders by becoming our eyes and ears when we are not there. Strongly recommend that family and friends have a clear understanding of the patient's diagnosis and our plan for their care.

Investing In Comprehension
Patients want to understand two things:

- Process: First, they want to understand how things will work. It's the health care provider's responsibility to inform them of next steps in their care. How and when they will be moving from triage to the treatment room. How long will waiting for lab results take? If they need to be admitted, how long will waiting for admission take? To medical providers, these steps seem obvious and logical, but to someone who is unfamiliar with the practice of medicine, it can all be a maze. Our job is to reduce patient anxiety by guiding them through the process of what to expect. We should give them a step-by-step process and help them understand why there may be some delay.

- Results and Diagnosis: Second, patients and their families want to understand their examination results and medical diagnosis. Do not use words such as *cholecystitis*, *diverticulitis*, or *choledocholithiasis*, without defining them. Patients might pretend that they understand these medical terms because they are too embarrassed to admit otherwise. What they really want to know, in clear and simple terms, is what their diagnosis and plan of care is. Explain this to them in a manner they understand and in turn they will be able to explain it to their family members without the help of a secondary medical translator. Remember that this is true regardless of the education level of the patient. Even patients with experience in the medical field need their diagnoses explained in layman's terms. This is because once they become a patient, they are often scared and cannot be expected to function as both a provider and patient simultaneously. Clear, concise communication is always critical.

Why Does The Patient Experience Matter?
Increased compliance = better outcomes.

The data shows that patients who have positive interactions with their healthcare providers are more likely to follow the advice given and adhere to the plans for their care. They are more likely to stop harmful habits, take their medicines, and not skip follow up appointments. This means they are less likely to bounce back with heart failure, a stroke, an MI (Myocardial Infarction) or worse.

Less Likely To Be Sued

Several studies consistently show that patients and their families do not initiate lawsuits against healthcare providers who communicate well and who explain medical matters in language that makes sense to both the patient and their families. This fact alone should be motivation to engage with this book.

Good For The Hospital, Better For The Staff

The experiences that a patient has in a healthcare facility will determine whether or not they recommend the facility. A positive experience usually leads to positive recommendations, new patients for the facility, improvements in the fiscal health of the hospital, resources to purchase state-of-the art equipment, retention of good employees by offering them raises and bonuses, and staff hires for understaffed facilities.

Improves Job Satisfaction

There are several studies that show an increase in staff satisfaction when providers have a positive experience with their patients. Staff satisfaction translates into providers who are more likely to enjoy their work, and consequently remain in practice for a longer period of time.

It's The Law

Finally, the Affordable Care Act of 2012 tied Medicare reimbursements to patient experience. Healthcare systems with high patient satisfaction scores are reimbursed at a higher rate, while underperforming facilities are penalized.

WHO COMPLAINS ABOUT PATIENT CARE?

Patients often complain about poor communication with their healthcare providers, including difficulty in understanding medical lingo, feeling rushed during appointments, or not having their questions or concerns adequately addressed.

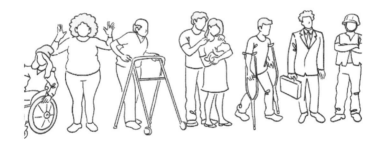

The Patients

In a similar fashion to any customers of any other industry, patients voice their discontent when their expectations are not addressed or adequately met. Patients complain about many things, including being unclear about their diagnostic test results, uncertain about their treatment plans, or uneducated about the process of medicine. Overall, patient complaints stem from a lack of communication or miscommunication between provider and patient. These communication missteps can be verbal or non-verbal.

Friends and Family

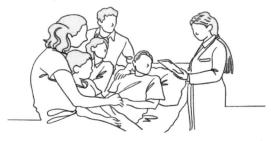

Friends and family are the patient's trusted companions and close relatives. Some members of this group might be present with the patient at the consultation or hospital visit. Some might only appear behind-the-scenes to support at the patient's home, in the neighborhood, or over the phone. These individuals who are highly influential to the patient will likely be involved to some extent in the patient's care and should be treated like the valued assets that they are. They are often privy to information needed by the medical team as they assess differential diagnoses. Remember that patients are often discharged into the care of a friend or a family member. I strongly advise that the patient's treatment plan be explained clearly to this support group. The feedback we receive from them in our satisfaction surveys will very accurately reflect back to us what they noticed about the way in which care was delivered to their loved ones.

Non-English Speakers

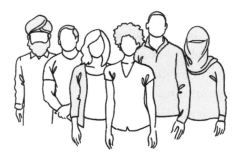

In the United States over 163 languages are spoken. Patients who come to our healthcare centers may not speak English. Trying to unpack medical terminology for this demographic in their native languages can be challenging, even with a translator. Explaining a medical condition to these patients in English is a different type of challenge that can often result in confusion and frustration on their part. It is important to make sure that in these circumstances, adequate measures have been taken to ensure that the patient/provider communication is effective. Patients who fail to achieve clarity about their conditions during the visit will certainly express discontentment after the visit.

What Do Patients Complain About?

Poor Empathy:

- When patients consult with providers who exhibit poor empathy, their perception is that the provider does not care about them. This was a common complaint during the early days of patient surveys. Sadly, more than thirty years later, this complaint still shows up frequently.

Bad Attitudes:

- "I knew by the tone of her voice that she didn't want me in her hospital."
- "She was saying one thing, but her face was telling me something else."
- "I could tell that this was the last place that the doctor wanted to be."
- "I felt like I was being judged by the nursing staff for my decision to come to the hospital."

Waiting times:

- "I waited for hours to see the doctor."

- "I pressed the call button numerous times, and no one ever came."

- "I waited and waited, and no one stopped by to explain why I was waiting so long or what I was waiting for."

- "I wish someone would have kept me informed during my 7-hour wait."

Technical issues:

- "The nurse/the x-ray tech...did not know what they were doing."

- "My labs took forever to come back."

Pain Management:

- "It took hours for the nurse to give me my pain medicine."

- "I was still in pain when I left the hospital."

- "The doctor thought I was looking for drugs."

Poor Communication:

- "They never told me I had a heart attack/cancer/a broken bone."

- "They never told me my lab results/who to follow up with/the side effects of these medicines/what to look out for/that I was being seen by a Physician's Assistant/a Nurse Practitioner."

- "The doctor never came back to explain, the CAT scan/the x-ray/what was wrong with me."

Unmet Expectations:

- "I came in for an MRI. I did not get it, and no one told me why."
- "I was told by my doctor that I was going to get a CAT scan. Why am I not getting a CAT scan?"

Billing:

- "The doctor came in, saw me for two seconds, and charged me thousands of dollars."
- "The doctor did not even examine me, and he charged me a fortune."
- "I was never told I was going to be billed by the 24/7 urgent care center as if I was in an ER."

Poor Team Communications:

- "They never told my primary care/heart/lung doctor that I was in the hospital."
- "The nurse told me I had one thing; the doctor told me I had something else."
- "The kidney doctor told me one thing; the lung doctor told me something completely different. Who should I believe? Who should I trust?"

IMPROVE THE PATIENT EXPERIENCE

The Right Disposition:

Before you enter the patient's room, put yourself in a place where you can be enthusiastic, welcoming, and sympathetic. The person behind the door you're about to walk into might be in a very vulnerable place, and they will pick up the nonverbal cues you may not even be aware that you are presenting. They might be feeling scared, out of control, and they may be imagining all sorts of worst case scenarios about their condition. These patients are looking for reassurance, hope, and a treatment plan that they can be optimistic about. What they do not need is a provider whose body language or facial expressions are off-putting or condescending.

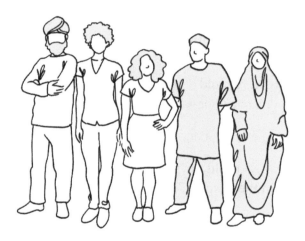

Cultural Awareness:

Familiarize yourself with the customs and traditions of the most prevalent cultural groups in your practice area. This knowledge can make all the difference in your communication strategies. For example, in some cultures children must not look adults in the eye, and authority figures (like a provider) must not be questioned. Information about cultural groups can really smooth things over during your consultation with individuals from these groups.

Some cultures are very free with physical contact and use it as a fundamental part of relating and connecting. In other cultures, individuals would be offended if touching occurred if respectful permissions were not first sought. Learning about the social norms of your patient population will be viewed as a powerful sign of respect, which builds rapport between the provider and the patient. Even more importantly, it builds trust, which motivates patients and their loved ones to adhere to the plan of care.

Respectful Service:

Under 30 minutes is the accepted quality service goal. If you know you are not going to be able to treat patients within this timeframe, let them know. Patients will wait if they are respectfully asked to. Yes, they would rather not wait. But they are there because they know the interaction they are going to have with you will be valuable, and the information you give them will be trustworthy.

Appearances:

Appearances say a lot about our professionalism. Patients and their families appreciate clean scrubs, professional attire, and lab coats.

Readiness:

Always be prepared. Have everything you need close-by. Keep your stethoscope, penlight, and tongue depressor handy. Maximize your time with the patient by eliminating any unnecessary processes.

Respect:

Address your patients as Mr., Ms., or Mrs. unless they tell you otherwise.

Eliminate Bias:

Many people knowingly or unknowingly carry biases. The biases may be towards ethnic groups, political parties , social classes, or even sexual orientations. Be very clear that biases do <u>NOT</u> belong in the hospital or medical office. Actually, they don't belong anywhere. Strive to get rid of them. Consciously or subconsciously, they will seep into your conversations with your patients. And when the cat is out of the bag about your bias, you will have damaged your trustworthiness, your brand, as well as your organization's brand. That may be catastrophic.

ENTERING THE PATIENT'S ROOM

Knock on the Door:

If there is a door, knock before you enter the patient's room. Unless there is an emergency, knocking is the courteous and respectful thing to do.

Busy Patient:

If the patient is busy on the phone when you knock, ask them if they would like you to come back in a few minutes. We have to remember that patients have lives outside the hospital, and sometimes non-medical emergencies (such as arranging child-care) do come up.

Apology:

If the patient has been waiting for a long time, apologize immediately. Don't blame anyone else and don't make excuses. An apology is a recognition that the patient's time is valuable. It has the power to placate a potentially angry patient, and to set up a healthy dynamic between the two of you. If you know the wait time will be longer than expected, have a team member notify the patient so they can plan accordingly. They may need to make alternate plans to have their kids picked up, pets fed, or even get coverage for work. Remember that patients have active lives outside of your facility.

Introduction:

No Healthcare provider should ever walk into a patient's room without announcing who they are and their role in the healthcare center. It's common courtesy and knocking on the door helps to orient the patient as they prepare to meet you. When you enter, a typical opening line could be along the following lines: "Hello, I am a Nurse/Resident/Xray Tech/ Anesthetist from the Pediatrics/Cardiology/ Surgical/Gynecology Department."

Inclusion:

Acknowledge and welcome everyone accompanying the patient. Make eye contact and ask about their relationship to the patient. By acknowledging the patient's entourage, you are making them your allies and creating a safe place for them to share relevant and potentially valuable information about the patient's medical history.

Inappropriate Questions:

Many providers begin their interaction with the patient by asking them the following question: "Why are you here?" This is a tone deaf question. Imagine going to your favorite hotel or restaurant and being asked, "Why are you here?" Some questions put the patient and their party immediately on the defensive and may discourage them from sharing critical information. Another inappropriate question often posed when a patient goes to the Emergency Room is, "Do you have an emergency?" This question is condescending because it implies that the patient can tell whether or not they are having a medical emergency.

Patients come to our healthcare centers looking for help. A respectful way to start the interaction is by asking, "How may we help you?" This question acknowledges the patient's need for our help and indicates our team's willingness to help them in any way we can.

Technology Devices:

iPads and other computer devices can take away from the interaction with the patient. The patient may perceive that the healthcare provider is disinterested or not listening. If you absolutely have to use a device, limit its use to a few minutes during the encounter, and never consistently for a long period of time. Tell the patient what you are doing on the device. For example, you might say, "I am checking your medical history and reviewing your medical records." Or you can ask, "Do you mind if we take some notes on the computer while you are talking?"

Proximity:

After entering the consulting room, move within two feet of the patient and step away from the door. If you stay close to the exit, you may convey the impression that you would like to leave, rather than stay with your patient. If you are further than two feet away from the patient, it will be harder to carry out the consultation in a conversational style or with a normal tone and volume of voice.

Sitting or Standing:

While the data does show a perception of increased time spent when the healthcare provider is seated, in the ER I normally stand. I only sit down when I have to deliver devastating news to a patient. In those cases, I typically get within two feet of the patient and place my left hand on their shoulder intermittently to connect with them. Remember, what matters here is your body language. It is not only what you do, but also how you do it.

Visual Cues:

Whether you are seated or standing, the patient will take visual cues from you. Your face, vocal tone, and body language all communicate as articulately as actual words. Your goal should be to activate visual cues that tell the patient the following: "I understand, I empathize, and I will help."

Listen:

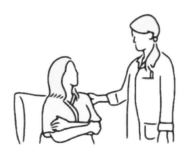

Listening can be a very difficult process for providers, mainly for two reasons. First, they are busy, and have many other patients waiting for them to see. They want to move as quickly as possible. Second, providers will be tempted to interrupt the patient if the information being relayed is not relevant or helpful to their differential diagnosis. Providers must make a concerted effort to listen. Firstly, interrupting too often can lead the provider to jump to conclusions about a diagnosis, make the wrong diagnosis and jeopardize the patient's health outcomes. Secondly, inattentiveness and interruptions can bias the patient against your care recommendations. After all, you couldn't possibly know what's wrong with them because you didn't listen to them when they were telling you about it!

Involve the Family:

If the patient is able to share their concerns, start by listening to them. However, do not forget to invite the family to share their own concerns or their version of the events that led to the patient coming to your healthcare center. As we know only too well, sometimes these two different perceptions of the same event can be completely different. Remember, these individuals could be helping to manage the patient's care after they leave your healthcare center. If that is the case, you want to make sure they are included in every aspect of the patient's care unless the patient says otherwise. Involve them!

Relate:

Patients need to know that doctors are human beings first and healthcare providers second. We can convey this by finding commonalities in non-medical things such as family and sports. When you engage your patient in conversations about the things that matter to them most, they feel more comfortable with you, and are more open about their medical problems, and will be more likely to adhere to the treatments you prescribe.. Most importantly, they will find you relatable and likable, and they will be more inclined to trust your judgment.

THE PHYSICAL EXAMINATION

Permissions:

Examining someone is a privilege, and the process is not always comfortable for the patient. Make a point to respectfully seek permission from patients, especially those who may be grappling with abuse. This directive includes children.

Do a Physical:

Patients often complain that they were not examined during their visit or that their health care providers did not even touch them. It should be standard practice to do a physical exam on every patient even if the diagnosis is already known. Patients and their families are suspicious when clinicians arrive at diagnoses without physically touching them. They see the physical exam as an integral part of the medical interaction. When we fail to examine our patients they think that we perhaps do not care enough, that we have not done our jobs well, and that we are not searching hard enough for the critical clue that may positively impact their diagnosis. The climate is such that patients now pay a larger share of their medical costs than ever before. When providers do not perform the physical exam, patients feel that they are not getting their money's worth.

Verbalize the Examination:

Tell the patient what you hear and feel. "This is your appendix, your gallbladder, your lungs are clear, your heart sounds fine." Why? Because doing so adds value to the medical visit. It helps correct misinformation acquired from friends or the Internet. It gives the patient information they can hold onto and take home with them. From a clinical standpoint, it may even help in the diagnosis.

Pain:

Let the patient know if a procedure or test to be performed might hurt. It psychologically prepares them for the experience.

Family members:

If the patient is an adult, ask them if they want family members present during their physical exams. Whether a family is present during the physical exam or not is completely up to the patient. *Always* ask permission when examining personal or private areas of the body.

THE PLAN OF CARE

Communication:

Tell the patient what to expect (the next step, the next tests, the next healthcare provider recommended) in SIMPLE terms - in a manner they can digest and explain to their family members who are not in the medical field. The process of medical care may be routine to us, but it is a very complicated maze for our patients. They, alongside their families, need our guidance navigating this process.

The Patient:

Involve the patient and their family in the plan of care you are recommending. Give them opportunities to weigh in, to share their thoughts with you, and to feel like they are an active participant in their own care. If they expected something other than what you are proposing, offer them a chance to discuss those expectations with you.

Medication and Side Effects:

Explain to the patient which medication you will be prescribing and their potential side effects.

Family and Friends:

Be sure to ask EVERYONE in the room if they have any questions. The quiet ones may be thinking something they are not sharing. Sometimes the quiet ones are the primary caretakers. Create an environment that encourages questions and opinion sharing. Presume that you are being recorded. Presume that once you leave the room a phone call will be made to a family member or a friend in the healthcare field. Some loved ones may already be on the phone. With the approval of the patient, have them turn on the microphone so the party on the line can hear what you have to say.

Time Commitment:

Tell the patient how long their tests will take and how long the entire visit will be. Always overestimate the time commitment because the healthcare environments can be unpredictable. It's important to remember that patients and their families have lives, obligations, and plans for the day. Patients are less anxious when they know how long the wait will be.

Be Accessible:

Tell the patient that you are only a phone call, an email, or a few steps away. Reassure them that if they have any questions, they can come and find you or they can send a message through the nurse. Let them know this applies to family members involved in their care as well. Doing this tells the patient that you are accessible, available, that you want to help, and that you are willing to help.

Elevate Coworkers:

Speak highly of every member of your team, especially if they are present. This instills trust in patients about your entire healthcare operation and shows them that their care team is united in their purpose to provide you with excellent care. It also gives your team members a lift and reminds them of team aspirations to surpass patient expectations.

Re-evaluate:

As you wait for labs or studies, re-evaluate the patient by including them in your Physician Rounds. Rounding is associated with a decrease in patient falls, patients leaving AMA, patients leaving without being seen, and the use of call lights. During re-evaluation, ask the patient about their initial complaints or new information? Are they worse? Better? Do they have new complaints?

Labs:

Check on pending lab work or imaging studies. Ask the patient and their family whether or not recommended studies have been done. If the studies are delayed, explain these delays without blaming other departments or staff members.

Team Communications:

Report any discussions you have had with anyone involved in the care of the patient, especially with their current physicians or any physician or specialist who will be taking care of them while hospitalized.

RESULTS AND DISPOSITION

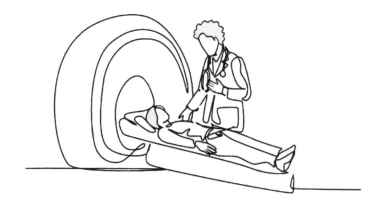

Labs and test results discussion:

When medical test results are discussed with the patient, the terminologies must be defined, clarified, and transmitted in layman's language. Providers often use medical terminology without explaining what the words mean. To the patient it is like someone speaking French to them when they only speak English. It will be incomprehensible. Medicine is very complicated. Find a way to simplify the medical terms to ensure patient understanding. They, in turn, will be able to relay their diagnosis to friends and families without having to call on their medical person for a better explanation. One technique I recommend is to sit down before the patient discussion, and to write down the medical diagnosis in simple layman's terms. Memorize what you have written and use it over and over in your practice. Before long, it will become part of your vernacular. When it comes to lab results, make sure to share with the patient what the norm is vs. what their results say, and what that therefore means for their diagnosis. Do not use general statements such as "everything looks good." Be very specific, especially if the patient was concerned about a particular aspect of their physiology, i.e., your kidneys are functioning well, there are no signs of infection, you did not have a heart attack....

Visual Aids:

Just like medical terminology, medical concepts are very difficult to conceptualize. Patients and their families always appreciate help in bringing abstract medical concepts to life. This can be accomplished by using visual aids. These can include drawings, using medical models, or videos.

Disposition:

If the patient is going to be admitted to the hospital, they need to know their diagnosis, as well as the results of their labs and other studies that were conducted. They need to know what will happen next, in terms of who will be managing their care while in the hospital. Be sure to share this information with all of the medical staff taking care of the patient. If the patient is sent to the Emergency Room, you will not be able to tell them how long they will have to wait for a room, as this is always unpredictable. However, you can keep them updated about the process and progress, which is information they will very much appreciate.

Transfer of Care:

A recommended option to sign a patient out to another health-care provider is to take the new healthcare provider to the patient's room to introduce them. Give the new provider a brief history of the patient's current medical issues including physical exam results as well as lab and study results. Include information about what is still pending and about the current plan of care. Speak highly about the incoming healthcare provider to alleviate any fears and anxieties the patients and their families might have about the impending change. I like this method of transfer because it is personal, and it allows for another visit to the patient by the outgoing healthcare provider. It also allows the patient to gain important information about their condition, especially if any misinformation was passed on from one healthcare provider to the next.

The other option is to perform the "sign out." This happens away from the patient, usually at the nurse or physician station. This method is more prone to errors that can be detrimental for the patient. It has more potential for false or incomplete information to be conveyed from one provider to another.

Regardless of the method that is utilized, always ensure that the patient and their family know about the transfer. Always make sure that the new provider, the patient, and the patient's family members all know what the current situation is, what is pending, the plan of care moving forward, and who will be taking over their care. Finally, always speak highly of the incoming healthcare provider to mitigate potential anxieties and fears.

THE DISCHARGE PROCESS

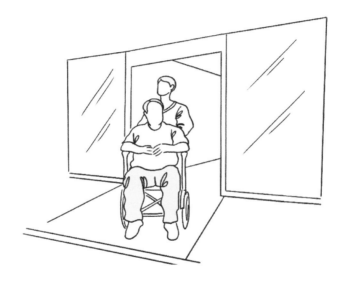

Information:

Everyone involved in the patient's care must know that the patient is being discharged. Give the medical staff necessary information about the post- discharge plan of care. Explain the plan in layman's terms to the patient and to their family. You may need to ask the patient to explain back to you their understanding of the plan you have outlined. Following this process will help expedite the discharge process, reinforce discharge instructions, and ultimately reduce readmissions.

Discharge Instructions:

Discharge instructions need to be given by the physician, nurse practitioner, or physician assistant, and should be reinforced by the ancillary staff. The following questions need to be addressed before discharge: What is my patient's diagnosis (if they have one)? If they don't have a diagnosis, what is known at this point about their condition? What happens if they get worse? Who will they follow up with, and when? What if they cannot get an appointment? What medicines will they be going home with, if any? What are their side effects? Will those new medicines interact with their current daily ones? What should they do if something goes wrong? Always end the discharge instructions with your patient by asking, "What questions do you have?"

Contact Information:

Every patient, and their family and friends, must go home with a means to contact the healthcare provider. This contact information reassures the patient that they will be able to call on you should questions, concerns, or unexpected new symptoms arise. Explain when you'll be available to address any questions or concerns. Based on my experience, very few patients actually call. The ones who do often have valid clinical questions or concerns.

Post visit phone calls:

Patient care does not stop when a patient leaves our facility. Post-visit phone calls should occur in the case of patients you are clinically concerned about, or who would benefit from some extra reassurance. These calls can also help smooth over fractured relationships with patients who may have poor experiences during their medical visits. The calls can be short, and yet can have a profound impact on the patient. Callbacks can also benefit the provider. It creates opportunities for them to correct misdiagnoses or change a false perception from the last visit. Do remember that patients can have bad outcomes after they leave healthcare centers.

Anytime:

When patients are leaving our healthcare facility and thank me, I like to reply by saying, "Anytime." It is a reminder that my healthcare center team and I are always ready to help. This open door policy is particularly helpful if that patient takes a turn for the worse.

SPECIAL CASES

The Hallway Patient:

Sometimes emergency rooms are so busy that patients actually end up in the hallway. In situations like this, it's important that the provider team make an extra effort to respect the patient's privacy. Always speak in a low tone of voice especially when discussing personal matters such as sex or abuse. Privacy is especially needed when discussing sensitive lab results. If overcrowding is an issue, provide the patient with privacy during the physical exam by using a sheet, a screen, or by temporarily moving them into a room. Finally, round on these patients frequently.

The Angry Patient:

Patients get angry because their expectations have not been addressed. When I see angry patients, the first thing I do, after introducing myself is apologize for whatever it is they are angry about. I listen to their complaints to find out what their expectations were, and how they were not addressed. Always acknowledge the patient's anger and frustration. Do not get angry. Do not minimize the patient's complaints. Do not cast blame on others. Admit wrongdoing and outline the steps that will be taken to remedy the problem. Follow up with a call to check on the patient and update them on the resolution of the problem. Give the patient your name and phone number and invite them to revisit your healthcare center.

The Demanding Patient:

Before walking into a demanding patient's room, understand that you will need to spend some extra time placating their concerns. Patients with unrealistic demands typically have underlying reasons for their discontent. These reasons may be centered around a misunderstanding of medical facts, or they might revolve around misinformation. Identify that reason. Once the medical concern is identified, educate the patient on the best practice processes for the issue. Provide follow up if needed.

The Patient with substance use disorder: "Drug Seeker"

"Drug addicts" are not in your health care center to insult your intelligence. Do not be offended by their presence. They have a medical condition: addiction. Be firm, be courteous, and be honest when interacting with them. Be upfront, but do not call them drug addicts. When discussing their chronic use of pain medicines, use the phrase, "dependent on pain medication." Do not let personal bias lead you to assume that a user is always an addict. Finally, patients who are chronic pain medicine users do have real medical problems that need care. You can easily miss those medical emergencies if you are blinded by personal bias.

The Patient In Extremis:

When a patient is in critical condition, invite their family and friends to be at their bedside. This may be the last time that these loved ones get a chance to interact with the patient. If you are resuscitating a patient, have the family at the bedside and explain to them what is happening to the patient. If you have to stop resuscitation measures, make that decision with the family. If the patient unfortunately does not make it, be the first to offer condolences, and take time to answer any questions that friends and family may have. Be tactful and sympathetic and offer your contact information for questions that may arise after they leave.

Change your mindset about communicating things you "would never come to the Emergency Department, the hospital, the office for"

- "I would never come to the hospital for this!"

- "She came in here for that?"

These are commonly used expressions in medical circles. However, we providers must refrain from passing judgments on our patients' decision to visit our healthcare centers. The difference between us and the patient is the obvious fact that we have medical knowledge. So, we are able to assess the potential gravity of a medical condition where our patients cannot. Another fact to keep in mind is that we all have different comfort levels with pain and our physiology.

Patients with Sickle Cell Disease:

Sickle cell disease is painful. Some patients with sickle cell do become dependent on pain medicine. This is not at a higher rate than the general population. Avoid getting worked up when we see these patients. Create a systemwide protocol to manage them. That protocol must be consistent throughout the health-care organization.

Discharged Patients:

Care does not stop when your patient and their family leaves the hospital, the office, or the urgent care. Bad outcomes can and do occur after discharge. So, we must do our best to minimize such outcomes by providing the patients with prompt follow-ups, our contact information, and by calling them at home to check on their medical status.

OTHER FACTORS THAT IMPACT PATIENT EXPERIENCE

Exhaustion:

Providers who work too many hours and too many consecutive shifts will get exhausted and will make mistakes. This is an administrative, a personnel, and a personal question. The provider and the administrators must be able to assess the number of work hours or the number of consecutive shifts that puts a provider at burnout risk. When does overwork start to negatively impact a provider's relationship with his patients, his family, or his coworkers? This is a very important question both for patient and provider safety, and you'll find most providers know their limit. They all have a number. What's yours?

Patience: Do not be offended

Do not be offended when patients or their families demand that specific studies or procedures be conducted. They have a reason and it's a provider's job to find out what prompted their request. So, instead of being offended, be patient and be tolerant. Talk to the patient and their family members and try to find out what's triggering these demands. What are they concerned about?

Do not be offended when a patient comes in with a complaint that you would never dare see a doctor about. We all have different comfort levels with pain or symptoms in general and behave accordingly.

Unreasonable Provider Expectations:

Just like patients, providers have expectations as well. We want a staff that is responsive to our needs. Test results turned around at lightning speed, and patients who will follow our medical advice to the letter. We may manage our expectations better if we can keep in mind the social, professional, and personal challenges facing our staff, our labs, and our patients. It is worthwhile to take a moment to pause, and to factor in people's real life challenges.

Inconsistency:

Use consistent patient engagement principles to treat every single patient and their family even when swamped. As patient load increases, and as more and more tasks are asked of us, we might revert to bad habits and maybe cut some corners with the amount of time we should spend with the patient. Recognize the benefits of sound patient engagement and make the choice not to reduce our interaction with the patient and their family. Remember that the right interaction with patients and their families not only makes clinical sense, but it also helps to decrease the number of future bounce backs, readmissions, phone calls, and meetings. Be consistent about the choices we make for our patients.

Imbalanced Team:

The patient-centered practice strategy starts with the head of the healthcare organization. This must be reinforced throughout the practice by individuals who have both direct and indirect contact with patients. If one part of the organization is rendering exceptional service and the other is not, an imbalance is created. Unfortunately, the negative experience will be the one that is remembered at the end of the patient's visit.

Quiz: How Can a Patient Be Satisfied?

6. Which of the following is not required for patient satisfaction?:

   A. Comprehension

   B. Expectations

   C. Giving the patient whatever, they want

   D. Participation

   Answer: C

7. A patient who is given whatever they want, including pain medications, is always satisfied with their experience.

   A. True

   B. False

   Answer: B

8. The two main things that a patient wants to comprehend are their results/diagnosis and:

   A. Their treatment plan

   B. The medical process

   C. Their costs

   D. Latin medical terminology

   E. What type of pain meds they will get

   Answer: A and B

9. Which of the following is not an outcome of a positive patient experience?

   A. More recommendations and referrals.

   B. More likely to be sued.

   C. More likely that a patient follows advice.

   D. Medicare reimbursement is higher.

   Answer: B

10. Studies indicate that healthcare providers remain in practice longer when they have increased job satisfaction.

    A. True

    B. False

    Answer: A

11. Overall, patient complaints stem from a lack of:

    A. Diagnosis or misdiagnosis.

    B. Time management during the office visit.

    C. Communication or miscommunication.

    D. Training among office staff members.

    Answer: C

12. Which was the most common complaint 30 years ago that still appears on patient surveys today?

    A. Technical issues

    B. Inappropriate billing

    C. Excessive wait times

    D. Lack of empathy

    Answer: D

13. Understanding that some people were taught not to look an adult in the eye, or not to ask a doctor any questions is all part of:

    A. Being culturally aware

    B. Looking professional

    C. Having the right disposition

    D. Addressing the patient with respect

    Answer: A

14. Everyone's time is valuable, even if they are not a doctor. A service quality goal should be to see patients within:

    A. 15 minutes

    B. 30 minutes

    C. 1 hour

    D. 2 hours

    Answer: B

15. No healthcare provider should never walk into a patient's room without announcing who they are and their role in the healthcare center.

    A. True

    B. False

    Answer: A

16. Which of the following questions is the most appropriate to ask a patient when first greeting them during an office visit?

    A. What is your emergency?

B. Why did you come here today?

C. How can we help you today?

D. None of the above are appropriate questions.

Answer: C

17. Which nonverbal communication should be avoided when engaging with a patient during their appointment?

A. Looking them in the eye.

B. Standing close to the door/entryway.

C. Standing or sitting close.

D. Leaning forward and giving your undivided attention.

Answer: B

18. Information gathered from attending family or friends may influence your diagnosis or tell a different story than the one shared by the patient.

A. True

B. False

Answer: A

19. It is important to ask for permission to physically exam a patient when:

A. The patient is a child that can verbalize an answer.

B. Examining any adult of the opposite sex.

C. You suspect a patient may have been abused.

D. Answers A and C above.

Answer: D

20. Your plan of care for a patient should include:

A. Communicating the plan to the patient in a simple manner (in a manner that can be shared to a person who does not belong to the medical field).

B. Involve the patient by asking for feedback and their opinion.

C. Involve any family or friends that will be caretakers and supporters.

D. All the above should be included in the plan.

Answer: D

21. True or False? Establishing and managing a patient's expectation is a major factor in the plan of care and promoting communication.

A. True

B. False

Answer: A

22. Studies indicate that rounding while patient's wait for the results of labs or studies to return correlates with:

A. A decrease in patients falls and leaving without being seen.

B. A decrease in patients using the call button.

C. Both answers A and B above.

D. None of the above answers.

Answer: C

23. One technique to communicate a diagnosis in layman's terms is to write it down on paper and then practice it over and over to avoid complicated medical terms when you are giving that diagnosis to a patient.

A. True

B. False

Answer: A

24. When performing a "sign out" transfer of care AWAY from the patient, which of the following is not part of the process?

A. The outgoing provider must notify the patient and their family that they are leaving.

B. The outgoing provider must review the plan of care moving forward and who will take over.

C. The outgoing provider must alleviate any fears the patient has concerning the incoming provider.

D. The patient and family must have the ability to correct any misinformation given by the outgoing provider to the new provider.

Answer: D

25. All the following are true of patients preparing to be discharged from the hospital or emergency room except:

A. The provider must explain the post discharge plan of care.

B. The provider in charge of the patient's care must avoid the patient and their family at any cost

C. The provider may have the patient and family repeat back their understanding of the discharge plan of care.

D. The provider must ensure that all the staff, patient, and family know the patient is going home.

Answer: B

26. Which of the following questions must be answered by the healthcare provider while reviewing discharge instructions?

A. What is the patient's diagnosis?

B. What were the laboratory and study findings?

C. Who does the patient follow up with? What if the patient is unable to follow up?

D. What are the side effects of medicines the patient is taking home?

E. All the above questions must be answered.

Answer: E

27. True or False? A post visit phone call to a patient with whom you had a poor interaction during the medical visit can give you an opportunity for a "do over" and provide you with a different insight into their behavior.

A. True

B. False

Answer: A

28. Which of the following is recommended when interacting with an angry patient at the hospital or ER?

    A. Apologize for whatever they are angry about and listen to them.

    B. Pass blame for the issue onto another department.

    C. Point out that they have the facts wrong and correct them.

    D. Refer them to another provider since they are unhappy with your staff.

    Answer: A

29. True or False? Biased assumptions that a patient is a "drug addict" may result in a medical emergency for that patient.

    A. True

    B. False

    Answer: A

30. All the following are true of patients with sickle cell disease, except:

    A. It is important to create a systemwide protocol to manage patients with sickle cell disease.

    B. Patients with Sickle cell have a high rate of addiction to pain medication which is higher than non-sickle cell patients.

    C. It is important not to jump to conclusions when attending to patients with sickle cell.

    D. The systemwide protocol to manage these patients must be consistent within the organization.

    Answer: B

MANAGING EXPECTATIONS

Anxiety:

A hospital stay can cause extreme anxiety for patients. Most people are not accustomed to the constant beeping pumps, moaning patients, or the calling out of orders. When a patient asks, "Am I going to die?" reassure them and calm their anxiety. In those circumstances I might say, "I am so glad you came in to be evaluated today. These symptoms/your condition could be dangerous if not addressed, and there may be a risk of death. But let me assure you that you're in the right place, and everyone in this facility is here to help you. We have all the tools to help you as best as we can, so I am really glad you came in today."

Transparency:

Whenever I evaluate a patient, I like to start our initial encounter by managing expectations. Transparency is key. After completing my history and physical I tend to end the conversation by saying something along the lines of, "I am concerned about a,b,c, so we're going to run *tests x, y, z* to rule them out. I can't promise that you will leave with a diagnosis, but my immediate concern is to ensure nothing dangerous is happening to you. That being said, symptoms may change so we would like to watch you for a few hours to make sure your symptoms are controlled."

Time:

In a world of same or next day delivery, our patients expect the medical process to be the same. This is especially true for newcomers to the healthcare system. The question, "why does it take so long" is a common refrain in our system when it comes to medical appointments, lab results, or study results. Some patients try to circumvent the system by going to the Emergency

Room, only to find that the services there can only address part of their concerns. Unfortunately, most medical diagnoses require a workup which can take hours to days.

Once a plan of care has been established, it is important to explain it to the patient along with the expected timeframe to complete our work up (always overestimate). We must be open about the potential curve balls that may delay the work up, and what can or cannot be done to avoid them. I always like to emphasize to the patient that the end goal is to get to the bottom of their symptoms, and to come up with a definitive diagnosis so we can get them on the road to recovery.

Definitive Diagnoses:

"I don't know" are words that healthcare providers are not comfortable uttering, because it implies an admission of ignorance. But admitting that we do not know is part of being transparent, and it takes away the misconception that doctors "know it all." Those of us who have been in practice for a while can testify that we know a lot about medicine, but there is still a lot more that we do not know. It is important that patients understand the limitations of our physical exams and tests. After going through the results of their current workup, I am completely comfortable telling patients if we still cannot explain their current ailment. The worst thing you can do in this scenario is make up a diagnosis. If you do that and you are found out, you will lose the patient's trust and respect, and you put yourself in legal jeopardy.

Scope Of The Workup:

Some patients leave the ER feeling like they "were checked for everything" Some patients leave the ER feeling like they were "checked for everything." I always jokingly wonder which Emergency Room checks for everything.

In the ER, I hear similar broad statements from patients about their primary care physicians, cardiologist, or other providers. This claim is highly unlikely.

When a study or lab test is ordered for a patient, it is our responsibility to detail the exact purpose and limitations of those tests to the patient and their family members. General comments such as "your labs are ok" can cause confusion. Avoid using general terms when discussing lab and study results. Instead use specific terms such as: "Your kidneys are working fine." "There are no signs of infection." "There are, however, signs of heart attack or stroke...."

Expectations From Family Members And Friends:

A significant portion of the patients that come to your facility are referrals from a family member, friend, or even from a search engine like google. Some of those patients are very upfront with the fact that someone else's bad outcome (their brother had a heart attack or a stroke) is the reason that pushed them into visiting the healthcare center. As we address the patient's clinical condition, we must dispel any judgment about the reasoning that led the patient to the healthcare facility.

After the medical interview, the first thing the patient will do when they leave the room is call whoever sent them to your facility. They will relay their perception of the interaction, the information you shared with them, including the plan of care or the clarification of any misconceptions.

Quiz: Managing Expectations

31. If a patient asks, "Am I going to die?" during a hospital stay, an appropriate response would be:

    A. Tell them that you are glad they came in to be evaluated.

    B. Downplay communicating any risk of death.

    C. Explain that they are in the best place with the best tools to help them.

    D. Answers A and C above.

    Answer: D

32. Which statement is true regarding expectations about time?

    A. Some patients may go to the ER to try and get things done faster.

    B. Most medical diagnoses require work up that may take hours or days.

    C. Explain the (realistic) expected timeframes to the patient for work ups.

    D. All the above statements are true.

    Answer: D

33. When managing expectations around a definitive diagnosis it is completely acceptable to tell a patient that you do not yet know why they have a current ailment, and that you are still evaluating to gather more information.

    A. True

    B. False

    Answer: A

34. Rather than telling a patient that "everything is fine" regarding test results, it is much more informative to explain exactly what was tested, why it was tested, and the results of that test.

    A. True

    B. False

    Answer: A

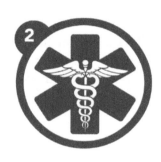

THIS, THAT, AND THE OTHER.

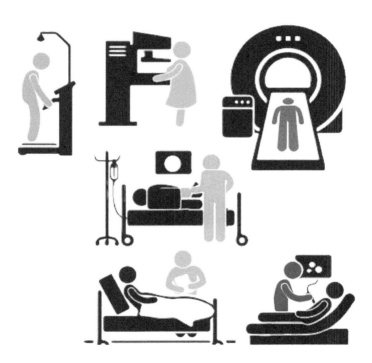

AFTER THE PATIENT GOES HOME

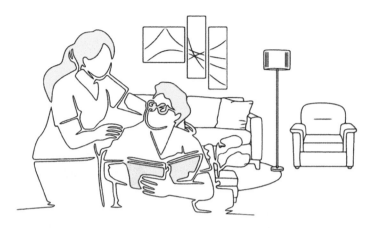

Follow Up After The Visit

After reviewing the ER medical data with the patient, I usually tell them something along the following lines: "We are giving you the name of a doctor. We want you to call tomorrow and make an appointment to see them. The work that we have done today tells us that you will need to see a specialist to address your current medical problems. If you are unable to see the specialist, please call me, or come back to the ER."

Business Card

Every patient discharged gets my business card. The business card is always accompanied by the dates and times I will be available to answer questions or concerns. How often do patients call me? In my 13 years of practice, maybe one call per year. Some of these calls have been lifesaving and have helped prevent any legal entanglement.

Calls

There are some discharged patients I call, and they fall into two categories. In one group are the patients who may have had an unsatisfactory hospital experience. In the other group are the patients about whom I am still clinically concerned, and who opted to go home.

PROVIDER CALLBACK: WHO DO I CALL BACK? WHEN? WHAT SHOULD I EXPECT?

Who to call?

- Patients you are medically concerned about
- Patients who were reluctant to go home or that you felt needed more reassurance
- Patients with whom you felt you had a less than desirable initial medical encounter.

When?

- 2-3 days after seeing the patient

What to expect?

- Your own reluctance: Being reluctant to perform call-backs is normal because no one wants to be judged
- Your nervousness: Being nervous during the first few calls is completely normal
- Brevity: Most calls take less than 1 minute
- The impact: Patients absolutely appreciate hearing the voice of a Physician who cared for them a few days ago

- Disparities: Don't be surprised by the disparity between what you said and what the patient heard

- Resolutions: Patients who leave your facility upset will be highly impressed by you taking the time to call and check up on their medical health.

What not to do?

- Don't take negative comments personally. View them as learning opportunities

- Don't limit your calls to the patients who will likely give you a positive response.

Chart Documentation

- I would include an addendum to the patient's chart detailing your conversation with the patient.

Callback Script

- Identify yourself and the facility you are calling from

- Identify the patient by name to verify identity

- Ask the patient if this is a good time for this call

- Ask them how they are doing/feeling? Are they better, worse?

- Inquire about filling of any prescriptions that they received, and if they had any of the potential side effects

- Ask them what questions they still have

- Provide any counsel about changes to their plan of care, if needed

- Thank them for their time, and remind them that you are available for questions.

Example:

Hello, this is Dr Jones from Woodrow Wilson Hospital. May I please speak with Mrs. Goldstein?

Hello Mrs. Goldstein, I am the doctor who saw you in the Emergency Room a couple of days ago

Is this a good time for you to talk? *Patient answers. Physician responds accordingly*

How are you feeling? Patient answers. *Physician addresses any problems*

Are you better, worse? Patient answers. *Physician addresses any problems*

Have you taken your medicines? *Patient answers. Physician addresses any problems*

Are you having any problems with those medicines? *Patient answers. Physician addresses any problems*

Have you called Dr. Smith to schedule your follow up appointment? *Patient answers. Physician addresses any problems*

What questions do you have? *Patient answers. Physician addresses any problems*

Thank you for your time!

I will be at the Woodrow Wilson Hospital on Thursday from 7am to 3pm If you have any questions or concerns, please give me a call.

Quiz: After the Patient Goes Home

35. Every patient that is discharged from a healthcare center should get the healthcare provider's business card, contact information along with the dates and hours they will be available for calls or to return calls.

    A. True

    B. False

    Answer: A

36. Providers should call certain patients 2 to 3 days after discharge if:

    A. They are medically concerned about them.

    B. The patient was reluctant to leave the healthcare center.

    C. They feel the patient had a suboptimal medical experience.

    D. All the above answers are reasons to call.

    Answer: D

37. Any comments made during a patient's call should be recorded in their chart, whether their condition has changed or not.

    A. True

    B. False

    Answer: A

38. The following should be included in a callback script, except:

A. Ask the patient if they have any questions or concerns.

B. Counsel any recommended changes to the care plan.

C. Ask them not to come back to your healthcare center if a new medical issue arises.

D. Always identify yourself and the facility you're calling from.

Answer: C

WHY?

Questions We Often Get From Patients and Suggested Answers

These answers can be used after a complete physical exam and related work up.

Why do I still have chest pain if my tests are negative?

We hear your concern. That is why we have checked for a heart attack, blood clot, collapsed lung, infection in your lungs, and water around your lungs. All those tests, thankfully, turned out negative. I can assure you that you do not have any medical problems that can cause immediate harm to you. The pain in your chest will require more advanced evaluation by a specialist and could possibly be due to irritation of your chest wall or something related to your stomach. We can prescribe medication for the pain; in case it is related to chest wall irritation. We will also give you the name of a specialist to follow up with so they can look into the other possible causes of your chest pain. When you call the specialist, please tell them I referred you. As you wait for your appointment, if your symptoms get worse or you develop new symptoms, I want you to call me, or come back to the ER.

Why does my stomach still hurt if my tests are negative?

We hear your concern. But let me assure you that we have checked for infections, blockages in your belly, kidney problems, and low blood count. All those tests, thankfully, turned out negative. At this point we have ensured that you have no medical problems that can cause you immediate harm. The pain in your belly will require a more advanced evaluation by a specialist, but we will give you some medicine for it as you wait to see the specialist. We will also give you the name of a specialist to follow up with, so they can look into the other possible causes of your belly pain.

When you call the specialist, please tell them I referred you. As you wait for your appointment if your symptoms get worse or you develop new symptoms, I want you to call me, or come back to the ER.

Am I miscarrying or not?

Note to providers: When you respond to this question, please do so with empathy.

Based on the tests we have done today, what we can tell you for certain is that your baby is in the right place. Unfortunately, the status of your baby right now is not optimal for a safe long-term pregnancy. The complications will require more advanced evaluation by a specialist. We would like to refer you to an obstetrician so they can further look into the issue. When you call the obstetrician, please tell them I referred you. As you wait for your appointment, if your symptoms get worse or you develop new symptoms, I want you to call me, or come back to the ER.

Why do I still have this headache if all my tests are negative?

We hear your concern but let me assure you that we have checked for strokes, bleeding in your brain, infection in your brain, and cancer. You do not have a medical problem that can cause immediate harm to you. All those tests, thankfully, turned out negative. The pain in your head will require more advanced evaluation by a specialist. We will give you the name of a specialist to follow up with so they can look into the other possible causes of your headache. When you call the specialist, please tell them you were referred by me. We will also give you some medicine for the headache as you wait to see the specialist. As you wait for your appointment, if your symptoms get worse or you develop new symptoms, I want you to call me, or come back to the ER.

Why aren't you doing an MRI for my back pain?

You are correct, you may need an MRI of your back. In the emergency room, however, we have a specific set of criteria that we use to determine if an MRI should be done. Currently your examination does not require an MRI today. This is good news! It means that we don't think you are at risk of immediate harm from your back pain. Furthermore, if we did an MRI in the ER, it would not change the recommendations we are going to give you. We are going to provide you with some medicine to help relieve your pain. We are also going to give you the name of a back specialist who you will call to make an appointment. When you call the specialist, please tell them we referred you. As you wait for your appointment if your symptoms get worse or you develop new symptoms, I want you to call me or come back to our ER.

Why don't you check for everything in the ER?

In the Emergency Room we typically check for low blood count, kidney problems, infection, problems with the organs that help process food, bladder infection, heart attack, blood clot, and stroke. We do not check for everything. We check for conditions that can cause immediate harm to your well-being. There are a number of conditions that we do not look for that may need to be evaluated outside the hospital by your primary care doctor or a specialist.

Why can't I see a specialist?

Patients often come to our healthcare centers with the expectation that they must see a specialist in the area of concern. This is particularly common in the ER, but it happens often in outpatient primary care as well. It is important to quickly identify or proactively address that expectation. In the ER there are specific criteria we use to determine when to call a specialist to see a sick patient. I always explain those criteria while reminding patients that these specialists additionally work in the community and have their own practices. On the outpatient side, it is important that Primary Care Physicians (PCPs) develop a relationship with their patients so that patients know to come to them first with any concern. PCPs should emphasize that they can treat the majority of ailments without referring to a specialist. They should make it clear that if a specialist is needed, they will refer early and advocate for their patient every step of the way. A PCP is best positioned to put the whole medical picture together for their patients and can provide continuous care to patients throughout their lives.

Quiz: Why?

39. When a patient asks why they have pain if all the diagnostic tests indicate no problem found, the best course of action is to:

    A. Explain the outcome of the current work up and the conclusion from those tests

    B. Give the patient a referral to a specialist if needed.

    C. Prescribe medication as needed to reduce irritation to the problem area.

    D. Tell them to call you if they get worse or develop new symptoms while waiting to see a specialist.

    E. All the above are the best actions combined.

    Answer: E

40. Regarding a possible miscarriage, speak to the patient with empathy. Let them know that if they are pregnant and bleeding and their tests show the baby to be in the right place in the uterus, they are still at risk of losing the baby. Let them know that they need to be monitored regularly by their OB/GYN.

    A. True

    B. False

    Answer: A

41. If a patient expected an MRI during their ER visit and did not receive one, you should tell them that not requiring an MRI is good news because they are not in immediate harm from their back pain. you don't think the issue calls for an MRI to determine a plan of care.

    A. True

    B. False.

    Answer: A

CAVEATS

Approach to Pelvic Exams:

In order to test patients with complaints such as changes in discharge, abnormal vaginal bleeding, or to do an annual pap smear, we need to perform an invasive exam known as the pelvic exam. As with invasive procedures, we must prioritize the patient's comfort. First and foremost, make sure your patient is in a private room. Hallway patients who need pelvic exams should be placed in a private room.

I like to explain the procedure before I ask patients to undress in the following way:

"In order to properly assess your symptoms, I would like to perform a pelvic exam. If you have ever had a pap smear, it is very similar. We will work together to make this quick and painless. I will give you a few minutes to remove all of your clothes from the waist down. Once you've done that I would like you to position yourself at the very edge of the bed with your knees bent and feet together and let your knees fall open, like a butterfly. I will insert a device called a speculum that will allow me to see inside your vagina. You will feel this insertion as pressure rather than as pain. Once it is inserted, I will examine your cervix and take two samples. If needed, I will also perform a manual exam. I will insert two fingers into your vagina and press on your abdomen to feel for any pelvic problems. A nurse/ colleague will be present throughout the exam to ensure your safety."

As this is an exam considered uncomfortable to most, it is important to talk your patient through it. Always announce when you are touching the patient, such as, "This is my hand touching you" and "I am examining your external genitals." Before inserting or removing the speculum, ask the patient to take a deep breath. Reassure the patient that they are doing great. Afterwards, thank your patient, and give them time to readjust themselves.

Educate During The Physical Exam:

The physical exam is an opportunity to provide tangible information to the patient and to dispel any misconceptions. Many years ago, I started verbalizing my physical exam with phrases such as, "Your lungs sound clear," or "I hear an abnormal sound from your heart," or "This is where your appendix is located." and I find that patients really appreciate the information. When I verbalize pertinent negatives, their fears seem to melt away. Other patients appreciate the fact that their knowledge about their physiology has been augmented or redirected.

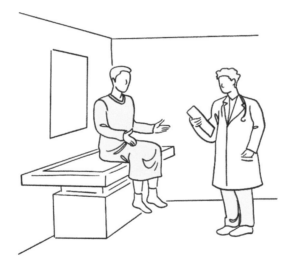

Altered Patients:

With patients who have had a mental status change, a history of dementia, inability to communicate verbally, intoxication or psychosis, make sure to gather information from the patient's family or authorized contact. Before reaching out to the authorized contact, confirm that they are in fact who you are looking for.

When I call, I tend to open the conversation along the following lines: "Hello, my name is *Dr. XYZ*, I am calling from *ABC Healthcare Center and I am looking* for the *family member of patient John Doe*. Is there a *family member of John Doe available? Do you have a moment to answer some questions about the patient?*" I tend to ask open ended questions because I am trying to gain an overview of the patient's general medical, surgical, and social history. If the patient lives alone, I would want to know if they have a caretaker, and what medications they take, including blood thinners. I want to find out the last time the patient seemed in normal condition, or allergies, and I would like to find out if the patient is medication compliant and if they attend their medical follow ups. Finally, I ask if the person I am speaking to will be accompanying the patient when they come to our facility. I always advocate for a family member to be at the patient's bedside for the benefit of the patient and the team.

Intubation:

In the Emergency Room we do not often have a chance to get a patient's loved ones involved in the decision to intubate. If it transpires that we do have the time to explain this very invasive process to a patient's loved ones, we should absolutely do so. These explanations to patients and families should be in language and terms that are clearly understood by family members, as they will undoubtedly be sharing this information with others. The reason for intubation, the actual process and alternatives must all be explained.

Potential Diagnosis Of Cancer:

After 13 years as a practicing ER physician, I am still uncomfortable walking into a room with medical data that points toward a new diagnosis of cancer. When delivering such potential catastrophic news to a patient and their loved ones, there are certain rules that I always abide by:

- Take a seat
- Get close to patient and family
- Be empathetic
- Be honest. e.g., Clarify what you can confirm in the moment,, what will be confirmed through further testing, and what other data will be provided by other specialists
- Console the patient and their loved ones by touching them. For example, placing a sympathetic hand on a shoulder is completely acceptable and encouraged
- Avoid getting into the expectation game. Do not speculate about how much time the patient has left to live.

Disclosure:

Once in a while we run into a family member who has the following request: "If it is bad don't tell [Patient]. Tell me first and I will decide if [Patient] should know." A loved one with the legal authority to make such a request is completely within their right to do so. The challenge arises when the person making such a request does not have legal authority and the patient is of sound mind. When the patient is able to decide who can know about his medical information, I explain that fact to the family members and I invite them to discuss who can or cannot know about the patient's medical information. When the family considers my challenge and they have a discussion with the patient, the issue is invariably put to rest.

Explaining Medical Laboratory Findings

At the end of the medical encounter when discussing results, we might say something like, "Everything looks good!" even if everything single thing is not perfect. Patients today have become more sophisticated and knowledgeable because of the availability of medical information on the Internet and because of increasing medical out of pocket expenses. I now tend to be more specific in my explanation of lab findings, and will use phrases like, "There are signs of infection;" "Your kidneys are working well;" "Your liver looks good;" "No signs of a heart attack at this time;" "No infection in your lungs;" "No signs of stroke."

I find that patients appreciate more specific information that they can take home with them and share with others.

Lab Test Results:

Always address any assumptions patients may have about the process surrounding medical lab tests and their results. A significant number of patients have the firm belief that the lab tests we order in the ER are tests for everything that could possibly be wrong with them. Address this misconception by specifically telling the patients the benefits and limitations of each lab test.

Education About Tobacco/Alcohol/ Drug Abuse

Whenever you take a patient's history, you will have to inquire about their relationship to drugs and alcohol. It is important when asking these sensitive questions that you do not come across as judgmental. Alcohol and drug abuse are addictions. Addictions are medical problems. Oftentimes, addictions co-occur with mental health disorders that often go untreated. Be kind. Be sensitive. You can consider asking these questions in the following way: "Do you mind if I ask you some questions about your use of alcohol or drugs?" I ask this of all my patients because it can affect your health, and also which medicines I prescribe for you." If the patient gives permission for the inquiry, you can begin by asking basic questions about whether they drink alcohol or use drugs. If they do, then you can proceed to use any of a number of validated screening questions for alcohol and drug abuse. If someone screens positive for alcohol or drug abuse, you should screen them for depression as well. Validated depression screening questionnaires such as the PHQ2/PHQ9 are good places to start. The most important thing here is to get information to help you make important diagnostic and treatment decisions about your patient's health. Your role is not to judge. Your role is not to get offended. Your role as a caregiver is to help patients open up about their ailments and their vices, and to seamlessly direct them to get help.

How To Use An Inhaler

An inhaler is useless if it is not used properly. It is important to coach patients with newly diagnosed asthma/reactive airway disease/COPD or multiple exacerbations about how to use inhalers and when it is appropriate to use them. **Controllers** (*budesonide*) are inhalers that should be used daily for maintenance. **Rescue inhalers** (*ipratropium*) are to be used during exacerbations. Prior to administering the puff, ask the patient to exhale all the way out. Then administer the puff, ask the patient to inhale deeply, and hold for 10 seconds before release. This is the proper way to administer an inhaled medication. Remind patients that it is important to rinse their mouth after using inhaled steroids to avoid oral thrush (a yeast infection on the tongue).

Moving Vehicle Collisions (MVCs)

Car accidents can be very scary for both patients and family members. It is important to prepare the patient for the soreness and pain that may come along with a deceleration injury. To this end I might offer an explanation along the following lines: "After an accident, it is very common to be sore, and even more so the day after and the days to follow. When your body takes a hit, , the impact can cause very tiny tears in your muscles, making them feel very tender. Drink lots of fluids, use ibuprofen like Advil or acetaminophen like Tylenol, and make sure to get lots of rest over the next few days."

Disposition to the ICU (Intensive Care Unit)

ICU admissions are another scary situation for patients and their family members. the language used to prepare them for this disposition should be well considered. In my practice I deliver this news by saying something along the line of, "Due to the severity of your symptoms/illness/disease, I recommend that you/your loved one be admitted to the Intensive Care Unit (ICU) for further management." The patient/their loved one might wonder why they are being disposed to the ICU rather than to a regular floor. You can choose to answer in the following way. "The ICU is an area of the hospital that has doctors and nurses specially trained to take care of the sickest people. These specialists are called intensivists. There are fewer patients in the ICU than on other floors of the hospital, so you will get very close attention from the doctors and nurses there."

COVID-19

COVID-19 is a sensitive subject in and outside the hospital setting. There are people who fear it and people who deny its existence. These opinions tend to be made along political party lines, but providers must stay impartial and leave politics outside of the hospital. I tend to ask every single patient their covid and flu vaccination status. I make sure to respond the same way regardless of the answer, "Are you COVID vaccinated? +/- booster?

Are you flu vaccinated? This season? "Okay, thank you." And continue on with my assessment. I make it a point not to entertain political statements or respond with blanket statements. All advice should be evidence based and supported by organizations like the CDC and WHO.

Intubation: Need For Intubation

Critically ill patients who are not properly oxygenating/ventilating/protecting their airway, may require intubation. I explain this in the following way to the patient/their loved one: "Your breathing pattern/level of oxygen in your blood/ability to think properly concerns me. I do not believe you will be able to keep going without some help. This help can be delivered by putting a tube in your mouth, through your windpipes, into the pipe that delivers oxygen to your lungs. We will put you to sleep prior to this procedure in order to prevent any discomfort. This process is called intubation. Once the tube is in, we will connect it to a breathing machine to help breathe for you, so you can rest. This type of machine is called a ventilator. It delivers lots of oxygen to your body and helps you heal. This is not often a permanent intervention. Most people come off the breathing machine once they feel better and the underlying issue is addressed or resolved." In cases where the patient is not conscious, I will give this explanation to their family members who are present.

Transfers:

Not all facilities have all the tools and personnel to meet every patient's needs. A provider should be able to recognize that a patient may benefit from being transferred to a more appropriate facility. I like to start with transparency and will typically offer an explanation in the following way: "We have reviewed your medical condition, and we have concluded that a transfer to a more advanced facility is your/your loved one's best option. If you agree to be transferred, a lot of pieces will begin moving at once. We will ask you to sign a consent form provided by the nurse, and then we will do the rest. I will call your family and explain this to them as well."

Natural Supplements:

I advise providers to tell patients that there is always a risk of taking any supplement that is not FDA approved. Patients also need to know that natural supplements can interact with medications and increase or decrease their metabolism. This can lead to a situation in which a prescribed medication regimen can become less effective, or more dangerous. Providers should always ask patients what types of medications or supplements/vitamins they take, and they should make sure the patient follows up with their primary care doctor to talk about what is right for them.

Adherence:

In a perfect world, all of our patients would take all their medications as prescribed and never miss a dose. Unfortunately, this is not a perfect world. It is important to discuss, educate, and acknowledge the patient's compliance status. I like to ask all patients questions like, "Which medications do you take? How often do you miss a dose?" Pose the question and your response in a non-confrontational tone. If a patient says, "You know doc, I take it when I remember to, but I'll admit I miss a few doses a week." do not reprimand the patient but praise them for their honesty and explain to them why it is so important to take their medications as directed. Ask patients about socioeconomic barriers that stop them from taking their medications as pre-scribed. When patients have to choose between buying food or buying medicine, they often do not choose to pay for the medicine. Ask patients about their struggles each time they tell you they are not taking their medication regularly. Be sensitive to this and link the patient with social services to help them get the resources they need. Try to avoid documenting the phrase non-compliant in the patient's chart. Instead, use non-adherent, or patient struggling to take medications as directed because.

Vascular Access:

Obtaining IV access can be challenging at times. Avoid sticking the patient multiple times. Use an ultrasound as soon as you determine that the patient's IV access will be difficult.

Quiz: Caveats

42. Which of the following are important aspects of pelvic examinations?

    A. Make the patient as comfortable as possible.

    B. Explain the process to the patient, then verbalizing each step as it is performed.

    C. Always have a female nurse or colleague present for the safety and comfort of the patient.

    D. All the above are important aspects.

    Answer: D

43. Which of the following steps are recommended when caring for a person with dementia or who cannot verbally communicate?

    A. Call members of the family or caretakers for the patient's medical history, and medication lists.

    B. Since the patient's wishes are unknown to you, you rely heavily on the family of the patient to find out their wishes regarding medical care and end of life questions.

    C. Ask open ended questions about the reason for the visit.

    D. Answers A, B and C above

    Answer: D

44. Which of the following is NOT part of the best practices when delivering a new diagnosis of cancer to a
patient.

   A. Take a seat close to the patient and family.

   B. Be honest about what you know and about what
   needs further testing and confirmation.

   C. Be stoic and detached from the situation so you
   maintain professionalism.

   D. Avoid discussions related to how much time the
   patient may have left.

Answer: C

45. True or False? Sharing information with a family member without informing the patient should only be done
if the family member has legal authority and the patient
is mentally impaired at the time.

   A. True

   B. False

Answer: A

46. Which statement is NOT true regarding discussions
related to drug or alcohol use with a patient?

   A. Drug or alcohol abuse tends to coincide with undi-
   agnosed mental health disorders.

   B. Anyone that screens positive for drug or alcohol
   abuse should be screened for depression.

   C. Recreational use of many substances should be
   reported.

D. Getting a patient to open up about their vices or untreated ailments allows you to direct them to get help.

Answer: C

47. True or False? Always advise patients to rinse their mouth after using any type of inhaler to avoid oral thrush.

A. True

B. False

Answer: B

48. Advice for a patient who has been involved in a motor vehicle accident include:

A. Informing the patient that they may be more sore tomorrow or the next day.

B. Informing the patient to drink lots of fluids over the next few days.

C. Advising the patient to take ibuprofen or acetaminophen as needed for pain and rest.

D. Advising the patient of all the above information.

Answer: D

49. Each of the following statements are true, except:

A. Advise patients that the ICU provides more specialized healthcare management than is available on the regular floors if they are averse to going to the ICU.

B. When possible, advise both the patient and their family about the need for intubation and how it works, prior to the intubation.

C. If a patient has not been vaccinated for COVID and verbalizes their beliefs against it, vehemently tell them that they are unintelligent and need to wake up.

D. Following an auto accident, inform the patient that microtears in their muscles happened during the accident and will make them sore until they heal completely.

Answer: C

50. True or False? Regarding supplements, inform patients that any supplement that is not FDA approved may interact with medications and decrease their effectiveness or present dangers.

A. True

B. False

Answer: A

51. If a patient informs you that they have not been taking their medication regularly, or as prescribed, you should:

A. Thank them for their honesty and explain why the medication is important.

B. Inquire as to their socioeconomic status and identify any barriers to obtaining the medications.

C. Refer any patient that is not taking their medications to social services for intervention.

D. Answers A and B above.

Answer: D

Moral Dilemma

Our profession exposes us to patients from all walks of life. We interact with sons, daughters, cousins, and grandparents; we meet individuals with a wide range of politics and religious beliefs, varying sexual orientations, diverse economic, professional, and social backgrounds. Most of the time, these interactions can be navigated relatively easily and safely.

I was recently asked some fascinating questions by Jonathan Munoz, a current medical student, that I felt would be beneficial to other healthcare providers: *"May I ask how you navigate patients who are/ have been incarcerated? Do you ever try to know what they were convicted of? I know it shouldn't change their clinical management, but does it change how you approach them behavior wise? What do you do when you go to see a patient who you know has done something horrible (i.e., child abuse). What about safety for you or your staff? "*

A great set of questions! First, I want to unequivocally state that the approach to all patients should *solely* be based on their clinical conditions. In other words, we should not decide whether to order a particular test based on a patient's social, political, or economic standings. Providers who modify their clinical approaches based on a patient's non-clinical attributes run the risk of making a potentially fatal clinical mistake. I must approach a financial supporter of the hospital the same way I approach the uninsured or the homeless patient. In fact, I do not ask patients about their insurance or financial means in order not to cloud my judgment. The only time I may ask about these issues is when the patient's social determinants of health may have influenced their presenting illness.

This 'blind' approach has to be maintained throughout every interaction with our patients. In an increasingly polarized society, health remains constant. Illness does not care about your political affiliation, sexual orientation, or religion. As such, we must be committed to making medical decisions that are NOT based on our personal feelings or led by our political or personal biases. I know first-hand how hard it is to exercise restraint. I was once punched by a patient and in that moment 'restraint' was the last thing on my mind. Luckily, I regained my composure by reminding myself that this patient was under the influence and was probably a completely different person without the drugs.

Safety is always a concern in the healthcare setting. We see folks who are at their absolute worst, physically, emotionally, and psychologically. My safety and the safety of my staff is paramount. That is why the gentleman in Bed #3 is in handcuffs, surrounded by three armed police officers.

I aim to keep my staff and myself safe at all times, while ensuring that every patient feels he or she is getting the best care possible. How is that accomplished in unpredictable or potentially dangerous situations?

1. When I walk into a room, I always make sure that I am situationally aware while at the same time placing myself within a caring distance from the patient (within two to three feet).

2. In potentially dangerous situations, I invite the security team to stand within arm's length of the patient

3. I always keep the patient's hands in sight while performing a physical exam

4. I check to be sure that anything that can potentially be used as a weapon is out of reach of the patient

5. I explain the plan of care in the same manner I would explain to all other patients: in a manner that is uncomplicated, respectful, easily understandable, and relatable.

And to Jonathan's question as to whether I want to know what an incarcerated patient is convicted of, the answer is *"No,"* because I do not want that information to cloud my clinical judgment.

Quiz: Moral Dilemma

78. Some patient information may cloud a provider's judgment if known, therefore it is best not to ask for details that are not related to their condition.

    A. True

    B. False

    Answer: A

79. Best practices for ensuring the safety of staff members when treating an unpredictable patient or when in a potentially dangerous situation include:

    A. Being situationally aware in a room and ensuring that anything that can be a weapon is out of reach of the patient.

    B. Ensuring that the patient's hands are in sight during a physical exam.

    C. Having a security team standing within arm's length of the patient.

    D. All the above best practices.

    Answer: D

Sexual and Gender Identification

Sexual orientation and gender identity are different things. Folks can be cisgender, meaning they identify as the gender that aligns with the sex they were assigned at birth. Cisgender folks can have a sexual orientation that is straight, lesbian, gay, bisexual, queer, or something else. This is their sexual orientation. Transgender folks do not identify with a gender that aligns with the sex they were assigned at birth. Transgender folks face particular marginalization, including folks denying that they exist. All folks under the LGBTQ category do not have the same experiences.

Do not assume anyone's pronouns or honorifics (Mr. or Mrs.). Ask folks how they would like to be addressed. Create an atmosphere where folks can feel comfortable sharing their pronouns. Each staff member should share their pronouns in conversation, so that a patient can feel safe to share theirs as well. Nametags can include those pronouns as well. This can create an open and sharing environment for the LGBTQ identifying patients and staff.

Do not assume things about people's lifestyles. People do not always want to be married, to have children, or to be religious. Do not assume every feminine presenting person has a male partner, or vice versa.

LGBTQ patients may have difficult experiences matching with the right caregiver. They may have had negative experiences with former caregivers and can find it difficult to trust medical providers. Like anyone, LGBTQ patients want to feel safe and cared for.

Gender non-conforming people and transgender people may have heightened anxiety and discomfort about their bodies. They may not feel comfortable getting undressed, or even removing an outer layer. Explain every step of the process and ask your patient what they feel comfortable with. Make sure spaces are in fact private.

Folks have agency and know their bodies the best. Accept what people say they need for themselves. Provide information, but don't question what folks say they want.

Quiz: Sexual and Gender Identification

T/F

Sexual orientation and gender identity are the same.

Answer: F

Cisgender folks identify with the gender that aligns with the sex they were assigned at birth.

Answer: T

Cisgender folks can be straight, lesbian, gay, bisexual, queer, or something else. This is their sexual orientation

Answer: T

Transgender folks do not identify with a gender that aligns with the sex they were assigned at birth

Answer: T

When dealing with LGBTQ patients assume anyone's pronouns or honorifics (Mr. or Mrs.). Do not ask LGBTQ patients how they would like to be addressed.

Answer: F

LGBTQ patients may have had negative experiences with prior caregivers and can find it difficult to trust medical providers.

Answer: T

Gender non-conforming people and transgender people may NOT have more heightened anxiety and discomfort about their bodies

Answer: F

Regarding LGBTQ patients and pregnancy tests be clear and provide a lot of information about the need and requirement of pregnancy tests.

Answer: T

Eight Hours...

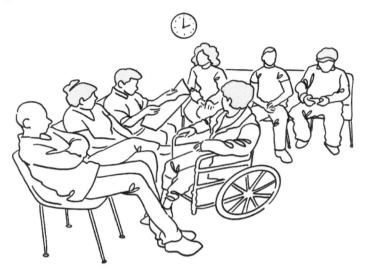

Can you imagine sitting in a waiting room for eight hours to see a healthcare provider? Would you patiently wait in your seat that long? Or would you be the type of patient who asks the triage nurse every five minutes when it will be their turn? If you have a friend at the hospital, would you be the type of patient calling them to find out if they can get you in faster?

I wonder which patient I would be. One thing I do know with certainty is that the healthcare provider had better be really good after waiting eight hours! "Good' for me as a patient means having my diagnosis explained to me in a way I can understand and relay to my family. 'Good' also means getting excellent care, empathetic counseling, and easy access to the services offered at the healthcare center.

We can deduce at least two things about this patient who waits eight hours to see a healthcare provider in my healthcare center.

1. The patient must know that the care he will receive is worth the wait. We are located in an area with many other healthcare centers that patients travel past as they make their way to our facility. Any of our patients could have easily traveled to a neighboring facility a few miles away to get the care they need. Yet, they did not.

2. As a provider, I feel flattered that someone is willing to wait that many hours to see me. I use the experience as a reminder that I must provide outstanding service, a worthwhile explanation and empathy.

When seeing patients who have been waiting for a long time:

1. Immediately apologize and explain the reason for the delay to diffuse any ill feelings. It is important to acknowledge that you value their time.

2. Update the patient often regarding the status of their labs and studies. Patients will forgive delays if they are kept in the loop, told the reasons for delays, and are updated on the status of their workup. Updating them allows them to adjust their plans outside of the healthcare facility.

3. At discharge, apologize once again for any and all of the delays they experienced.

Quiz: Eight Hours

80. True or False? A patient will only wait many hours to see a healthcare provider if that provider's service is worth the wait.

   A. True

   B. False

   Answer: A

81. If a patient has waited a long time to see a provider, it is important to:

   A. Apologize for the wait when you see the patient.

   B. Keep the patient updated about the status of work up results.

   C. Apologize for all delays when the patient is discharged.

   D. All the above are important.

   Answer: D

SECTION THREE
SPECIAL ATTENTION

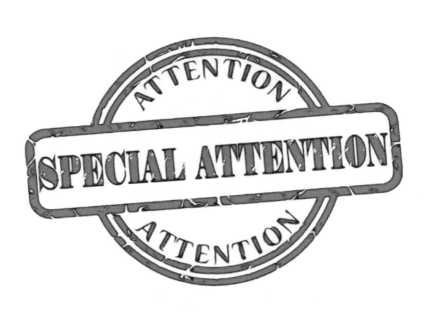

The Pediatric Experience

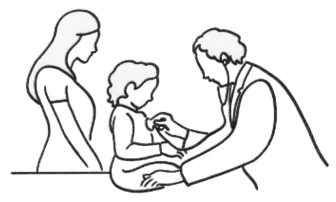

Seeing a pediatric patient requires all the skills discussed so far in this book and more. Why? Because a medical encounter that combines a worried and fearful parent with a sick patient who may or may not be able to communicate their symptoms, can lead to a very volatile situation. Both of these challenges must be adroitly addressed to diminish anxieties and maximize clinical outcomes.

Here are some general guidelines when seeing a pediatric patient:

1. Understand and address the parents' concerns. Parents fear the worst about their child's condition. Their concerns may be based on secondary or non-medical information. Take time to listen to their concerns, reassure them, and educate whenever there is a need. I like to assure parents that their child "is in the right place" and "we are going to make sure they are ok"

2. Remember to explain yourself to both the patient, assuming they are at an age they can understand, and the parents

3. Explain the process of the medical work up. This is very important. Children have significantly less patience and/ or ability to understand than adults. Parents usually have other matters in their lives that need to be tended to. Explaining the medical steps that will be required to look into the patient's complaints helps the parents understand and plan their day accordingly

4. Be sure to interview the patient, as long as they are able to verbalize answers

5. Prior to examining anyone under 18, ask for their permission

6. During the physical exam get to the eye level of the patient

7. Explain the physical as it is being performed

8. Let everyone know if something is going to hurt

9. If patients are unable to verbalize their concerns because of their age, or underlying medical conditions such as Cerebral Palsy, listen to their parents. Parents spend more time with their children than we do. If they tell us that something is wrong with their child, believe them. Sometimes the child may look completely fine in our facilities. Regardless, we would be wise to presume that something is wrong until proven otherwise

10. If at all possible, enlist the child's support by educating them about their condition. I have been repeatedly impressed by children's capacity to understand their medical condition and consequently take an integral part in their recovery.

Quiz: The Pediatric Experience

82. Which of the following is NOT a general guideline when treating a pediatric patient?

    A. Interview the patient if they can verbalize answers.

    B. Let everyone know if something is going to hurt before you do it.

    C. Leave the parents in the waiting room so the child can focus on you.

    D. Like with an adult, always explain the process in a way that the child will understand.

    Answer: C

83. True or False? It is completely acceptable NOT to share expected work up timeframes with concerned parents.

    A. True

    B. False

    Answer: B

I WANT A MEDICAL TEST!

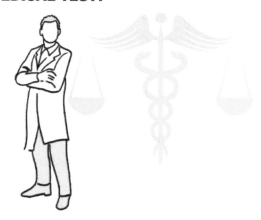

Sometimes, A provider has to determine the medical appropriateness of tests their patients may ask them to perform. How they respond may shape the impression the patient has of their medical services and may also have a significant clinical impact.

Here are some general guidelines on how to address these question:

Clearly understand why the patient wants that test. *Ask the patient for clarity. "Why do you think you need a CT scan?"*

It is very important to have a clear sense of why the patient wants that test. Their answer might be revealing: "To make sure I do not have cancer."

It is equally important to communicate our understanding of their goal in a clear, concise manner.

Do a complete physical exam:

Patients are more willing to accept our recommendations when they know we have done our due diligence by performing a complete physical exam.

Provide information about their medical concern:

Take time (yes, I know we have limited time) to educate the patient and their family about their medical concerns. Sometimes the request of a study is rooted in false information or misinterpretation of medical information. It is important to correct any misinformation in a non-judgmental manner.

Provide information about the Tests:

Patients often have partial information about the tests they are requesting. We must clarify and dispel any misinformation our patients may have regarding the tests we are considering performing. All risks and benefits must be explained, and the shortcomings of those tests must also be explained. Thus, the patient may be surprised to hear the provider's response: "A CT does not necessarily rule out cancer."

Avoid Discussions about Cost:

Bringing up the cost of imaging studies may give the false perception that the reason the test is not being done is to save money.

Quiz: Medical Tests

84. Explaining to a patient that every test has a significant cost associated with it is a perfectly sensible reason to justify not ordering imaging for their condition.

   A. True

   B. False

   Answer: B

85. The best approach for managing a patient's expectations when they request imaging that you did not intend is to:

   A. Refer them to whatever imaging they requested just to make them happy.

   B. Understand the patient's reasoning, address their concerns, and communicate your diagnostic goal.

   C. Perform a complete physical examination to demonstrate that you have done due diligence.

   D. Answers B and C above.

   Answer: D

Improving The Ancillary Staff's Experience

Can you check this EKG? Can you come to room 6? Code heart in room 21! Stroke alert in room 2!.Dr. Benson is on line 2 holding for you! The list of things that are being thrown at providers daily seems to never end. In the daily grind of our individual healthcare centers, it is easy to forget that the other members of our staff face challenges that may be different but might be just as difficult to manage. To make sure our patients are having the best experience, physicians and clinicians need to ensure that the ancillary staff is having an even greater experience. As you engage your staff:

- Be sure to know everyone's name: the nurses, the techs, and janitorial staff

- Show appreciation for their work through rewards and recognition in front of their peers. Do not hesitate to thank or compliment nurses, medics, environmental personnel, registration clerks, X-ray personnel, clinical pharmacists, and others on their accomplishments. They need it!

- Keep channels of communication open by encouraging the ancillary staff to share ideas, concerns, and disagreements about patient care. Cultivating such an environment can prevent medical errors and save a patient's life

- Think about each staff member's role and appreciate their crucial importance to our daily professional lives

- Remember that the ancillary staff delivers the majority of patient care.

- We must do some introspection. We must ask ourselves whether or not our behavior toward the ancillary staff is having a positive or negative effect on the care of our patients

- Personalize your interactions. Some ancillary staff members prefer a verbal reminder of the order placed in the EMR. Some do not. Find out their preferences

- Remain professional at all times; yet be friendly, and build rapport with the ancillary staff

Quiz: Improving The Ancillary Staff's Experience

86. Ancillary Staff handle most of the patient care in your organization, and they should be rewarded and recognized for their efforts in private so as not to embarrass them.

    A. True

    B. False

    Answer: B

87. True or False? Taking the time to know everyone's name on your ancillary staff roster demonstrates that you care about them and take an interest in their part within the organization.

    A. True

    B. False

    Answer: A

Engaging the Nursing Staff

The nursing staff is the lifeblood of medicine. They care for patients in a manner that physicians are not able, willing, or interested in doing. Having a great professional relationship with the nurses (and other members of the medical team) is crucial to achieving great patient care. There are a few tenets that I live by when working with my nursing staff:

1. Treat everyone with respect. We all know that nurses provide the majority of medical care. They spend more time at the bedside than any other provider. They should be acknowledged for all they do and deserve our utmost respect.

2. Invite them to share their opinion. As nurses spend most of the care time with the patients, their opinion is valuable. When we create an environment where they can share their views, it creates a powerful professional environment which leads to better patient care and outcomes.

3. Educate at every opportunity. Nurses are avid learners. Explain carefully and invite them to ask questions whenever an order is unclear.

4. Make their lives easier. In the ER, nurses may ask me to put orders in that should have been placed by the admitting physician. I understand that it helps the nurse when I do this, so I do. I grab pillows, chairs, or blankets for patients whenever I can. All those seemingly minor gestures deepen our professional bonds and engender mutual respect. It also sends a message to the patients and their families: their health is in the hands of a great team.

5. Celebrate them publicly. My nurses are the best nurses in the world. I make this very clear at the beginning of the patient encounter. It helps reassure the patient that they have the best team of people working on their medical issue, and it sets expectations for the entire medical team.

Quiz: Engaging the Nursing Staff

88. Guidelines for engaging with the nursing staff include:

A. Creating an environment where they can share their views.

B. Treating them with respect and acknowledging all that they do.

C. Educating them at every opportunity and inviting them to ask questions.

D. All the above are guidelines for engaging with nursing staff.

Answer: D

89. True or False? The nursing staff will appreciate your helping to make their lives easier by minimizing their workload and helping with small tasks that they would normally handle.

A. True

B. False

Answer: A

LESSONS FROM THE PANDEMIC

Patient Needs During The Pandemic

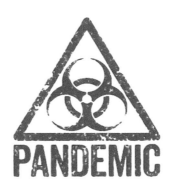

The COVID-19 pandemic put a lot of stress on our healthcare system and strained our professional and personal lives. Our patients need us more than ever, especially when conflicting information about the pandemic is still being shared with the general public by different news outlets. In our role as caretakers, translators, and educators we strive to meet the needs of our patients as they navigate the challenge of surviving the pandemic.

How do we do this?

1. Manage Stress: There are so many more things in this pandemic environment that can cause you significant personal stress. Take appropriate measures to ensure that you have the right disposition before coming to work. Don't take your issues out on your patients. They need us to do better.

2. Manage Bias: We all have personal views about this pandemic and the political echo chamber surrounding it.

Those views are our own and should be kept out of your facilities. Biases at your place of work will emerge during the medical encounter, and may lead to poor medical outcomes

3. Exercise Tolerance: Understand your patient's concerns. Some of them may be scared, anxious, or have an unclear diagnosis. They may be searching for information, and your job is always to provide and deliver that information in a patient and tolerant manner, in a way that they can understand and explain to others.

4. Involve Family: Keep your patient's family members informed. During the pandemic we changed our visiting protocol. As a result, a number of family members could no longer directly participate in the care of their loved one. That should not stop us from reaching out to family members who are outside of the healthcare center or at home, to acquire more medical information, provide updates, discuss plans of care, and enlist their help as our patients are discharged

5. Explain. Explain. Explain.

Provider Needs During The Pandemic

The patient's experience is heavily dependent on the provider's holistic wellness. Most of us have been under significant strain during the COVID 19 pandemic, trying to manage our professional medical duties as well as our concerns about our own personal health and the safety of our family members and our colleagues. Those additional layers of anxiety can negatively impact our interaction with our patients and their families. We can minimize the impact of this new layer of stress in the future by doing the following:

1. Minimize Exposure: Have a protocol in place to minimize exposing your family to the virus. After your shift, have a decontamination procedure in place at home, and be consistent about going through the procedure before spending that well-deserved time with loved ones. The last thing we want is to share an infectious agent with the people we deeply care about.

2. Mental Breaks: When you are not working, take a full mental break. The cycle of news regarding COVID-19 and its impact was nonstop at one point. Stories about colleagues who fell to the virus as they tried to heal their patients spread very quickly, and that grim outlook took its toll. Constant streams of negative news can impact us mentally and emotionally, to the point that we are pessimistic and apprehensive even with our patients. Take periodic breaks from the news cycle and the negative streams of pessimism. During your break, remind yourself of the importance of your role and the reasons why you got into medicine in the first place. Periodic breaks can help you refresh your spirits.

3. Support Colleagues: In times of dire crisis, we have to support each other more than ever. This pandemic was a new phenomenon, and it upended all aspects of our professional and personal lives. During a pandemic we need to support and engage with each other more frequently, checking in on all the members of our care team. 'All' means everyone from the physician to the custodian. -The COVID-19 pandemic has heightened the importance and impact of our interdependency.

4. Activity: Take a periodic break from medicine all together. What providers do every day is physically, emotionally, and mentally exhausting. I am a big proponent of having an activity outside of medicine in order to reset my psyche. Mine is gardening in my yard, and volunteering in Haiti. If you already have an activity that helps you to decompress, great! If you don't, please find one, and be intentional about making time for it.

5. Hold On: We are the wall. When you are feeling low, when things are tough, when you experience, doubt, fear, or apprehension, hold on. Remember that WE ARE THE WALL! And the wall must hold.

Quality Care **During The Pandemic**

The COVID-19 pandemic changed things drastically for the medical profession. But in all that change the fundamental premise of the patient-healthcare provider interaction remains constant. It is still based on the patient's need for clear, concise information, and the healthcare provider's clear and empathic response. How can we fulfill our part of this patient-provider contract when we have to grapple with new types of barriers like the masks, gowns, and personal fears of contracting the virus?

1. Tone: Our tone of voice matters now more than before. We are now wearing multiple layers of protective equipment. In most cases patients cannot see our faces or facial expressions. Consequently, they now rely on cues such as the tone of our voice to determine if we care, if we are angry, exasperated, in disbelief, annoyed, or impatient.

2. Body Language: We have to wear Personal Protective Equipment (PPE), but that means that patients are

unable to fully read our body language. Nevertheless, they will still look for clues there. We can communicate with our body by doing things like moving closer to the patient, standing away from the door, touching the patient, doing a physical exam, and by verbalizing the findings of the physical exam.

3. Calm Fears: PPEs are scary. Most patients are not accustomed to seeing healthcare providers in such garb. When a patient sees a healthcare provider coming at them with multiple layers of protection, they can experience anxiety, and may even question how bad their disease is. If we do notice that fear from our patients, remind them that our new dress code is for their protection, as well as that of everyone involved in their care.

4. Share Information: Providers will always be purveyors of medical information. Patients will always come to us with symptoms and expect us to translate those symptoms into a medical diagnosis. No pandemic can change that aspect of our work or detract from our ability to communicate with our patients and their families. Effective communication is achieved when information is transmitted from healthcare providers to patients in language that they can share with friends and family without the help of a secondary translator.

COVID-19 REMOTE FAMILY COMMUNICATION TIPS:

- Call the patient's family right after you first see the patient. That initial call can help corroborate the history, allay fears, fill gaps, and frame the plan of care

- Call the patient's family with ANY emergent updates as you wait for final disposition, labs, and studies

- Call the patient's family loved once or disposition has been established. Discuss pertinent labs and study findings in a manner that the family member understands, and can explain to others after you hang up

- Finish every call by asking if the family member has any further questions

- Offer times and dates that you will be available to answer questions, and provide a call-back number.

On Stage

Remember that we are always on stage:

- Keep your antenna tuned. Something that seems benign to you may truly be offensive to others, and may create a lasting perception of you, your staff, our healthcare system, and our medical field

- There is always someone listening whether we are aware of it or not

- Presume that your patients or their families are recording your conversations and interactions with them.

Quiz: Lessons from the Pandemic

90. During a pandemic it is important to minimize exposure to our family by ensuring that we have a decontamination procedure in place before spending that well-deserved time with loved ones.

    A. True

    B. False

    Answer: A

91. During a pandemic it is important to always stay focused on our healthcare profession to help as many people as possible, canceling personal time and devoting all our time to solving the problem.

    A. True

    B. False

    Answer: B

92. All the following are true in order to effect a positive patient experience during a pandemic, except:

    A. Body language and non-verbals no longer provide any communication since everyone is covered in PPE, so focus on what is said.

    B. Explain to the patient that the PPE is necessary for the safety of everyone, including themselves.

C. Patients still need to understand the process and the plan of care and must have them explained in a manner that they understand.

D. Answers A and C above.

Answer: A

93. True or False? When communicating remotely with family members of a patient with COVID-19, always end each communication by asking them if they have any questions that you can answer.

A. True

B. False

Answer: A

Relationships in Healthcare:

Few providers use the word 'relationship' when referring to their patients. Even fewer strive for a personal relationship with their patients. It absolutely benefits everyone concerned (patient, family, provider) if there is a humanizing element to support the medical consultation and treatment. This is especially true in the face of increasing clinical and clerical burdens, and the litigious environment we inhabit. A personal relationship with your patients and their families can enhance effective communication and help to achieve good clinical outcomes.

So, how do you ensure that the staff in your organization cultivates a professional yet personal relationship with your patients and their families?

Provider-Provider Relationships:

When I went to medical school there were no team building exercises. In fact, I would argue that the process of getting into medical school and medical school training pushed me to primarily rely on myself and to view my colleagues as competitors. In residency, the focus was on clinical management of patients. Team building exercises were not formalized and emerged only as a by-product of interactions with the ancillary staff and other specialists. My first team building exercise did not occur until I was pursuing my MBA. That is when I realized how valuable this approach could be to my work in the medical field.

The funny thing is that when you graduate from residency, you are magically expected to know how to operate smoothly as part of a medical team. This, without the benefits of any training about how to function well as part of a medical team and how to interact with other specialists, ancillary services, and non-medical staff to achieve good medical outcomes and support positive patient experiences. Not surprisingly, many physicians struggle with being effective parts of a medical team even though team relationships are crucial to the effective delivery of healthcare.

Codependency:

If you are a member of a healthcare team, you necessarily depend on your colleagues in the collective effort to provide exceptional care for your patients and their families. The physician depends on the nurse; the ultrasound tech depends on the physician; the anesthetist depends on the cleaning crew. There are multiple links of care around a patient and their families. Those links must realize, embrace, and find ways to improve and sustain co-dependence. Open, strong, and respectful bonds lead to better outcomes for all.

No Robots:

The daily grind of medicine means that sometimes members of your healthcare circle may behave like robots, churning out report after report, or delivering increasingly efficient services. But remember that they are not actual robots. They are human beings, subject to the same challenges and emotions as the next person. Part of your role as a team player is to keep open ears and eyes as you interact with your colleagues. This approach will help you pick up subtle clues that a team member may need some support. That support can be in the form of simply taking the time to listen to them, or asking a coworker about their day, or inquiring about a family member.

Engage:

You and your colleagues can leave a powerful imprint on the patient and family experience if your team members are in a good place of wellness. So, play your part in creating a happy workplace environment. Take the time to engage with everyone involved in patient care. Try to connect beyond your profession by sharing non-medical experiences and activities. 'Everyone' includes the cleaning crew, the techs, the nurses, the physicians, and the administration. Everyone!

The Provider-Patient Relationship:

When I was in residency, some of my attendings had a favorite saying: "treat them and street them." My colleagues and I understood that we would not be creating long-term relationships with our patients when we graduated out of residency. Some of the attendings believed that the care of the patient stopped at discharge, and that there was no need to establish a post-discharge pathway of communication with them.

Thankfully, things have changed somewhat. In today's medical environment the care we provide in healthcare does not stop at discharge. In fact, I would argue that what happens after discharge is the most important determining factor in a patient's road to improved health. It is the post discharge window that is most important in determining future health, readmissions , and skyrocketing healthcare costs. Rather than 'street them', we must remain engaged in our patients' care after discharge. Furthermore, we must establish and maintain a relationship with our patients and their families while they are physically under our care, and remotely after they have left our healthcare centers.

Benefits of Provider-Provider or Provider-Patient Relationships

- Improve patient care delivery
- Improve remote patient care (with physician not at bedside)
- Improve speed of care delivery
- Improve team functioning

- Improve team communication
- Increase likelihood of staff member sharing other issues
- Decrease staff turnover
- Improve staff morale
- Improve staff satisfaction
- Increase sense of belonging
- Improve patient care delivery
- Decrease number of unnecessary calls to Healthcare Facility
- Decrease bounce backs
- Less litigation

Necessary Components of Relationship Building:

- Acknowledgement by all parties that they are part of a team
- Acknowledgment by all parties of the roadblocks to team betterment
- Willingness by team members to learn more from/about each other
- An environment that promotes cooperation, a willingness to share, and support each other
- A team/healthcare center leadership that creates the appropriate engagement environment
- A team/healthcare center leadership that is forward thinking and engaged
- A team/healthcare center not stuck in the "ivory tower"

Quiz: Relationships in Healthcare

94. The co-dependent provider-to-provider relationship must foster team building and mutual respect for all members of the team at all levels and downplay competitiveness within the team itself.
    A. True
    B. False

    Answer: A

95. The benefits of forming strong relationships within healthcare include:
    A. Improved speed of care delivery
    B. Improved team communication
    C. Improved staff morale
    D. All the above benefits

    Answer: D

96. The components necessary to foster strong relationship building include:
    A. An environment that promotes cooperation and a willingness to share.
    B. Acknowledgement by all parties that they are part of a team.
    C. A willingness by team members to learn more about/from each other.
    D. All the above components.

    Answer: D

THE OTHER SIDE

Over the years, I have been privileged to have my colleagues and staff members entrust me with their health. I have treated nurses with cancer, physicians with diverticulitis or heart attacks, and even providers in abusive relationships presenting with psychiatric challenges. Some colleagues have referred their family members and friends to my care. Interactions with these patients often offer a glimpse into the private world of my colleagues, which in many cases is quite different from the public persona they adopt in the workplace. I appreciate being given a chance to learn more about my colleagues with whom I spend more time than my own family.

I've come to realize that many healthcare professionals are amazingly talented at pretending that all is well. I don't know if it is because we assume we must appear "better than the patient" or if we think we must appear "strong in front of our colleagues." We typically separate our professional and personal lives, but occasionally personal challenges spill into our professional space. And during such times, hopefully an astute colleague will notice something, lend an ear, or offer some counseling.

Keep a heart, ear, eye out for colleagues who may be going through profound personal challenges and pay attention to their level of engagement. If someone is less present, the reason may be personal. Taking the time to notice, listen and possibly offer advice or some form of resolution can lead to a professional win. Genuine care from and for colleagues can contribute to a great work environment. It can build collegial trust, rapport, and respect. It promotes open communication. And it ultimately leads to a better customer (patient) and family experience. The next time one of your colleagues is acting out of character, take a moment to inquire about their challenges. You may provide some temporary solace, or even save someone's life.

Quiz: The Other Side

97. If your colleague is struggling, underperforming, or uncharacteristically frustrated, showing empathy may provide them with some temporary solace, or even save their life.

    A. True

    B. False

Answer: A

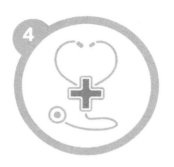

PATIENT SPEAK

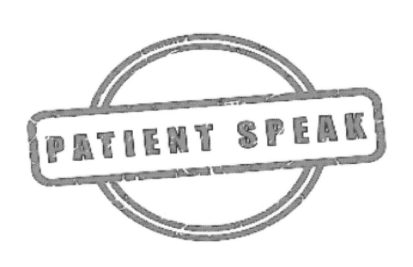

Preparing the patient for trauma assessment:

Always, always, always introduce yourself to trauma patients whose care you are involved in. I like to get close to the patient and say something along the lines of, *"Ma'am/Sir, my name is Dr ***. You were in an accident. There will be a lot of people touching you and it might feel overwhelming, but we are all working together to make sure you're okay. It's okay to be scared, but just know that we are here with you."*

Explain why you're removing their clothes. *"We need to cut your clothes off to get a thorough look at your injuries. We will use blankets to keep you covered."* Give words of encouragement. *"You're doing great."* Give them a warning before you change tasks. *"I am going to use an ultrasound, a type of camera, to perform an exam on your belly and check your organs. The jelly we apply to your skin will be cold, but it will give us a better picture. Next, we're going to roll you over to check your back, when the time comes, give yourself a big hug and let us do all the work. All I want from you is that you focus on where I am pushing on your spine and tell me if there is pain in that spot."*

Before performing an indicated rectal exam, you must explain to the patient, *"We need to perform a rectal exam, using a gloved finger, I need to check if you are bleeding internally and see if your spinal cord is damaged. It will be uncomfortable, but it will be quick and will give us important information. You will feel some pressure on your bottom and then we will be done. Once we complete our assessment and address your wounds, we will take you to the CT scanner (essentially a magnifying lens) to take pictures of the body parts about which we are concerned."*

Medications

Medications and Side Effects:

Every medication has the potential to cause some unexpected reactions, though not everyone gets them. Be sure to explain the following to patients, in detail: You can say something along the lines of, *"Here are some of the side effects you may have from this medicine. If you have those side effects please call or come back to our healthcare center."*

Medication Explanation:

Doctors often prescribe medications to patients without breaking down how those medicines work, or why they are important. The doctor might say, *"Your cholesterol is high so I will be starting you on a statin medication."* But the ideal statement should say, *"Your cholesterol is high. This means that you are at a higher risk of having a heart attack, a stroke, or liver problems. Diet and exercise are by far the best ways for you to lower your cholesterol and I will give you some tips about how to start a nutrition and exercise regime. But because you also have diabetes, and because heart disease runs in your family, it is important for me to offer you a medicine that can lower your cholesterol AND lower your risk of having a heart attack. This medicine is part of a class of medicines called statins. These medicines prevent your liver from producing too much cholesterol. You should still work hard at eating healthily and exercising every day. In fact, if you do this, we may be able to cut down on the dose of the cholesterol medicine, or even stop it altogether in the future. But it is really important that you take this medicine now while you are working on your lifestyle changes."*

Yes, it takes longer to do this, and time is something we do not have a lot of in medicine. However, if you explain it well the first time, your patients will be so much more likely to trust your judgment, take the medications, make lifestyle modifications, and, most importantly, live healthier lives. They will understand that the health choices they make, in combination with the medicines you prescribed, (if needed), are directly responsible for improving their health.

Studies

Abdominal CTs with PO Contrast:

This is a procedure that requires pictures to be taken of the organs in your belly. In order to get a good view and image of these organs, the patient must drink a liquid that will outline more clearly the relevant organs in the image.. This liquid will also lower the chances of us missing anything. After drinking, we will need to wait a certain amount of time before we take the picture, to ensure the liquid has traveled through your intestines. The whole process should take x number of hours.

CT (cat scan):

A CT scan machine uses an advanced camera to take very good pictures of any part of your body. It can even take pictures of your blood vessels to see if you have blood clots. A CT scan does expose you to radiation that can cause cancer later in life.

MRI:

An MRI machine is another type of camera that can take a very good picture of any body part. An MRI machine can also take a picture of your blood vessels to see if you have blood clots. However, an MRI does not expose you to radiation that can cause cancer.

Ultrasound:

Diagnostic ultrasound—also known as sonography—is when we use a special camera that uses sound waves to give us a look inside of your body. An ultrasound is used to perform many procedures. It can be used to place an IV, check on pregnancies, diagnose gallbladder disease, evaluate blood flow, assess the thyroid, examine breast lumps, and assess joint disease. It is virtually harmless. We can perform a bedside ultrasound to get a quick clinical picture. When we want a more detailed picture we can order a formal ultrasound, to be performed by an ultrasonographer in a different area of the hospital. This type of ultrasound will be read by a radiologist. An ultrasound gel is applied to the skin before starting the exam. This gel helps us get a clearer image of the body part we are examining. Ultrasounds can help us with information about fluids or blood in the belly after a trauma such as a stabbing or a gunshot wound to that part of the body.

X-Rays:

X-rays are cameras that take pictures of parts inside your body. X-rays can give us an idea of how badly a bone might be broken. But sometimes x-rays can miss broken bones. Moreover, they cannot show torn ligaments (string that attaches one bone to another). In other words, x-rays are not 100% accurate. You may have been sent for an x-ray scan by your doctor because of suspected broken bones. Even if the scan is negative, you may still have a broken bone or a torn ligament that was not picked up by the x-ray scan. In such cases you should talk to your primary care doctor or call a bone doctor so they can run some additional tests.

Incidental Findings:

Quite often while doing a CT Scan or an MRI we stumble across incidental findings. An incidental finding is something that was discovered while checking the patient for other issues. It is important to always maintain transparency, and to report these incidental findings to the patient. I like to print the results and hand it to the patient, suggesting a follow up with their PCP. For example, if n an incidental pulmonary nodule is appreciated on a CT, I might tell the patient, *"Your CT ruled out what we were looking for. However, there was an incidental finding - a spot/mass we noted on examination. This may very well be benign and not cancerous, but it's important that you follow up on it. Here are your results. Make sure to call your primary care provider right away and provide them with your result."*

Procedures

Family Members:

Always ask the patient directly if they would like their family member present during a procedure. However, it is up to you if the family member stays or not. If the family member would like to stay, I seat them wherever the patient would like them to be positioned. Sometimes, the patient requests that their loved one be placed close to them so they can hold hands and lessen their anxiety. Remember to ask the family member if they will be able to tolerate watching the procedure. I have had family members pass out during a procedure.

Foley Catheter:

A foley catheter is a tube that drains the bladder and keeps track of the amount of urine the patient has produced. Sometimes a foley catheter is needed to relieve an obstruction between the bladder, and the penis or vagina.

Incision and Drainage:

In infections like boils or other irregularities, fluid or pus collects in an area underneath the skin causing pain, swelling, and sometimes worsening infection. To relieve this condition the fluid can be drained by numbing the site, making a cut, and letting the site drain out. Sometimes, we put gauze in the area to diminish the risk of fluid re-accumulating and reinfecting the site.

Joint Aspiration:

Fluids tend to accumulate in the parts of the body in which there is inflammation or infection. Fluid can accumulate in any joint in your body. If the fluid needs to be tested or removed, we use a needle to extract the fluid. This is done after the area is cleaned and numbed.

Lumbar Puncture:

The brain and the spine are bathed in a liquid called the CSF (Cerebrospinal Fluid). This fluid has direct contact with the brain and the nervous system. As such, the CSF can be used to indirectly assess nervous system issues such as meningitis. A sample of that fluid can be obtained by inserting a needle in your low back after it has been numbed. That fluid can then be sent to the lab for analysis and to determine the best treatment plan.

Laceration Repair:

Laceration repair is one of the most common procedures performed at a patient's bedside. When there is a break in the skin (laceration), there is risk for complications of infection and scarring. We close lacerations to promote wound healing, to prevent contamination, and for cosmetic purposes. It is impossible to guarantee that there will be no scar, as with any break in the skin, there is a risk of scarring. If the cut is deep, we may need to close the wound in layers. We typically use absorbable sutures, which do not need removal as they will dissolve on their own. If non-absorbable sutures are used they MUST be removed by a professional within a time frame that varies by body parts. A local numbing medication (lidocaine) is applied to the site prior to washing out the wound to lessen any discomfort. This numbing medicine is similar to what they use at the dentist. The wound will be washed with saline (similar to water) before repairing your wound. After the repair is complete, bacitracin (an antibiotic ointment) may be applied to prevent infection. The sutures should be kept dry for 24 hours. If there are any concerns, including worsening redness, swelling, pain, or any pus-like discharge , the patient must return to the medical facility immediately to be evaluated for infection.

Explaining Antibiotic Effectiveness:

Antibiotics are a type of medicine used to treat infections. When the antibiotic is in your gut, some of it is absorbed; but by a germ/bacteria the rest comes out of your body when you pee or poop. Because some stay in your body and some leave, most antibiotics take a few days to work effectively. It is important to tell your doctor if you are not feeling better after taking an antibiotic for several days.

Sample Layperson's Language For Various Medical Conditions

We have taken the time to list the most common conditions encountered by providers and translated them into 'patient speak.' Use these explanations as a guide for communicating with your patients. You should modify the language to fit your speaking style. The goal is to engage your patients, to be empathic, and to convey the essence of the diagnosis and prognosis in a way that helps them understand their medical issues and take charge of their recovery process.

HEAD, EARS, EYES, NOSE, THROAT

Conjunctivitis:

Conjunctivitis is an infection of the white part of the eyeball. You can get infected by a germ (bacteria or virus). That germ could come from you, if you had a recent respiratory infection, or from someone else you came in contact with. The eye infection that you have can be given to other people very easily so make sure you wash your hands before touching anything or anyone. Conjunctivitis can be treated with medications such as antibiotics if caused by a bacteria.

Ear Infection (*Otitis Media*):

Your eardrum is at the end of the ear canal. Its job is to help you hear and prevent stuff from going deep into the canal. The space behind the eardrum can get infected and cause your ear to hurt. Usually, you get an ear infection when you have a cold, or soon after. Ear infections can be caused by bacteria or viruses. Ear infections are treated by antibiotics (if caused by a bacteria) and drops.

NEUROLOGICAL

Stroke:

Your brain controls everything that you do: walking, talking, swallowing. Different parts of your brain are responsible for those actions. For example, the back of your brain controls your eyes. Blood flowing to the brain allows those functions to take place. Blood flows through a series of pipes that we call arteries. When there is disruption to the flow of blood in those pipes in the brain, we call it a stroke. Sometimes a blood clot can cause that blockage and disrupt blood flow to the brain. We treat strokes by removing any blockage to blood flow in the brain.

Mini stroke (Transient Ischemic Attacks) (TIA):

A ministroke is when the blood flow to a section of the brain is blocked for a little while, and then the blockage goes away on its own. We know this because the patient's initial symptoms (cannot walk, talk, lift arm) go away and the patient reverts back to normal. Treatment of small strokes focuses on prevention of larger strokes, where the symptoms do not go away. Medications are aimed at preventing clogging of blood vessels.

Tissue Plasminogen Activator (TPA):

This is a chemical that we can inject into the patient having a stroke to help break up the clot that is stopping the blood from flowing to the part of the brain. This medicine has to be given within a certain amount of time from when the symptoms started. That medicine has some risks. It can cause bleeding in the brain and can worsen the patient's condition.

Brain Bleed:

When blood spills out of the blood vessels onto the brain tissue, it's called a brain bleed. Several conditions can cause the blood vessels to rupture: hitting your head, too much pressure in the blood vessels (hypertension (HTN), or a tear in the blood vessel wall. Brain bleed can cause symptoms similar to a blockage in the brain blood vessels. These symptoms include dizziness, difficulty speaking, difficulty walking, and one sided weakness.

PSYCHOLOGICAL

The Baker Act: (Involuntary institutionalization)

A mental health act enacted in 1971 allows involuntary institutionalization of patients for a maximum of 72 hours or until
patients are cleared by a licensed psychiatrist. In Florida, this is
called a Baker Act. The patients are usually not in a mental state
to understand the process. Once a decision has been made to initiate the Baker Act it is important to explain the process and consequences to both the patient and their loved ones. The patient
may ask, *"Why am I being Baker Acted?"* Answer: *"We have made
the decision to enact a Baker Act this time. We made this decision
because we have concerns that you are a danger to yourself and to
others. Our job is to ensure you are medically cleared for evaluation at a psychiatric facility. We will collect samples of both blood
and urine as well as any necessary imaging to ensure there are no
other underlying medical conditions causing this behavior. We will
have a staff member sit with you until you are formally admitted
or transferred to ensure your safety."*

Important questions to ask patients prior to initiating a Baker
Act are: *"Do you currently have any thoughts of suicide/ or wanting
to hurt yourself? Do you have a plan? Do you currently have any
thoughts of wanting to hurt others? Do you have a plan? Are you
hearing voices or seeing things that other people can't hear/see?"*

CARDIOVASCULAR

Myocardial Infarction: MI (Heart attack):

The heart is a muscle, and just like any other muscle in your
body it needs blood to work. That blood is brought to the heart
muscle by small pipes called arteries. When there is blockage in
one of those pipes, the heart muscle cannot pump the way it is

supposed to. This leads to pain in the chest, difficulty breathing, dizziness, and sweating. We know you are having a heart attack because the heart releases a panic chemical when it is not getting enough blood. When the heart is malfunctioning, its electrical circuit is also in trouble, and we can pick that up using a machine connected to your chest called an EKG. Heart attacks are treated by using medicines to open the clogged blood vessel(s).

Heart Failure:

The heart is a muscle whose job is to pump blood around the body. Just like any other muscle, the heart muscle can be come weak, fatigue. A number of conditions can cause the heart to become weak such as high cholesterol, diabetes, high blood pressure. When that pump weakens blood flow is diminished and fluid starts to back up. The first place it backs up into is the lungs. Heart failure can be treated with medications depending on the cause.

Pericardial Effusion:

The heart sits in a sac. Between the heart and that sac are spaces which can fill up with fluid. Fluid that fills that sac can be blood, associated with an infection, or fluid from cancer. The fluid around the heart can be removed by a surgical procedure.

Aortic Aneurysm/Dissection (tear in wall of aorta):

There is a big pipe(a large blood vessel) that carries blood from the heart to almost every part of your body. That blood vessel is called the aorta. The wall of that blood vessel is made up of several layers of tissue. Conditions like high blood pressure and habits like cigarette smoking can cause that blood vessel to have a bulge. That bulge is called an aneurysm. Those same conditions and habits can also cause a tear in one of the layers that make up the wall of that blood vessel. That is called a dissection. Just like any pipe that has a tear in its wall, the tear in the blood vessel wall can rupture and lead to a massive amount of bleeding inside your chest or in your belly. The bulge, or aneurysm, can be fixed by a surgeon before it ruptures.

Gangrene:

Your fingers and toes are warm and have their natural color because blood is able to flow to those areas and bring oxygen to them without any obstruction. If there is a drop in blood flow, or a complete blockage in the blood flow to your fingers or your toes, they will turn blue. If that blockage persists, the tissue in your fingers and your toes will start to die and turn black. That is called gangrene, which can be treated by medications and by an operation.

Hypertension:

When the pressure in your blood vessels is 140/90 or above, on two or more occasions, you have high blood pressure. High blood pressure is caused by a number of factors. The most common causes are salty foods and genetics (your mom or dad passed it on to you). High blood pressure is usually treated with diet (avoiding salt) and exercise. In some individuals, diet and exercise need to be supplemented with medications. If the pressure in your blood vessels remains persistently high, it can cause severe damage to your heart, your brain, and your kidneys.

PULMONARY

URI (upper respiratory infection):

The upper part of your respiratory system includes your nose, throat, and your windpipe. Sometimes that part of your breathing system can get infected by a germ (virus) causing you to have pain in your throat, coughing attacks, a runny nose, and fever. Treatment of upper respiratory infections focuses on addressing the symptoms associated with it.

Asthma Attack:

Asthma is a condition that affects your lungs and makes the tissue in your lungs more sensitive to certain irritants. When you have an asthma attack, you start to cough and have a hard time breathing. For people with asthma, things like cigarette smoke (whether you are smoking or someone near you is smoking), inhaled chemicals, dust from your house, pollen from flowers outside, and viruses can all cause a sudden inflammation in your lungs. That inflammation will cause an asthma attack, and that is when you have trouble breathing. You may even feel that you cannot breathe at all. An asthma attack is treatable with medicines that will reverse the inflammation in the lungs and allow you to breathe better. Asthma attacks can be prevented by regularly using an inhaler to control the inflammation in your lungs.

Pulmonary Embolism/Deep Vein Thrombosis (PE/DVT) (blood clot):

Blood flows through your body using pipes we call veins and arteries. Veins are responsible for carrying blood away from parts of your body to your heart. When blood moves slowly or stops moving, it can lead to the formation of a blood clot. A blood clot can be created in those veins and can diminish or even stop blood from flowing out of that part of your body. For example, a blood clot in your leg shows up as swelling of that leg – meaning that blood is having a hard time flowing out of that leg. There are a number of conditions that put you at higher risk of developing a blood clot. Blood clots are treatable and preventable by using medicine to thin the blood and ultimately break up the clot.

COPD/Emphysema:

Your lung tissue was built to be stretchy in order for oxygen to flow in and out. Nicotine damages the lung tissue and takes that stretchiness away. This leads to the lungs not being able to move air out of your body. This makes it hard to breathe.

Pneumonia:

Pneumonia is an infection of your lung that is usually visible on an x-ray. It is caused by a germ (bacteria, virus, or fungus) that makes its way to your lungs. You can get this germ when other people around you who are sick do not cover their mouths when they cough. You can also get pneumonia when the cells in your body that are supposed to defend you against pneumonia do not work properly. Things like smoking and diabetes can make it more difficult for the cells in your body to defend you from pneumonia. Pneumonia is usually treated with medications called antibiotics.

Bronchitis:

Bronchitis is an inflammation of the lining of your lungs. The inflammation causes your lung tissue to swell up, which leads to coughing, fever, and sometimes difficulty breathing. When you have bronchitis, x-ray results look normal; they don't show that you have pneumonia. Bronchitis is typically caused by a virus and treated by addressing the symptoms - like the cough or fever you experience. Antibiotics are not typically needed to treat bronchitis.

Pleural Effusion:

Your lungs are surrounded by a cover of tissue called the *pleura*. There exists a potential space between the lung tissue and that layer of tissue. When fluid enters that potential space, it is called a pleural effusion. The fluid around the lung can be removed by a surgical procedure.

Pneumothorax (Collapsed lung):

Lungs are like balloons filled with air and placed in a container called your chest. There is a space between your chest wall and the skin of the balloons (lungs). A collapsed lung occurs when air leaves the lung and goes into the space between the lung and the chest wall. That escaped air pushes on the lung and causes it to shrink. It causes symptoms such as difficulty breathing or pain in your chest. That condition is treatable by inserting a tube through your chest wall to allow that air - in the space between the lung and the chest wall - to escape.

GASTROINTESTINAL

Gastritis:

When you eat certain foods, drink alcohol, or smoke, the lining of your stomach can get irritated. Typically, the inflammation can cause pain after you eat or drink something that irritates your stomach. You can also have some vomiting with the irritation of your stomach. This condition can be treated by changing what you eat, and/or taking medications. We usually recommend following up with a gut (GI) doctor to keep track of this condition.

Stomach Ulcer:

Alcohol, bacteria, smoking and certain foods can cause irritation of the lining of your stomach. If that irritation continues for a long time, the lining of the stomach can break down, causing a small hole or ulcer to form. This condition can be treated by changing what you eat, and/or taking medications. Follow g up with your gut (GI) doctor to make sure that the lining of your stomach is healing.

Cholelithiasis (Gallstones):

Your gallbladder is an organ that looks like a pear. It is located on the upper right part of the belly. The gallbladder's job is to collect chemicals (called bile) and use it to help break down foods that we eat, especially fatty foods. The gallbladder can develop stones in it. The stones are made up of cholesterol which is found in high fat foods. The stones can make it hard for the gallbladder to work and can cause pain and vomiting. By decreasing the fat in your diet, you may be able to improve the belly pain and prevent vomiting. If changing your diet doesn't help the pain or vomiting, then you may need surgery to remove the gallbladder. There are no fast acting medicines to get rid of the stones. The main solutions are diet changes, or an operation.

Cholecystitis (Gallbladder infection):

Sometimes the stones in the gallbladder can cause it to become infected with a germ (bacteria). This is called cholecystitis. This infection of the gallbladder can be treated with an operation to remove your gallbladder, and with medicines to treat the infection. You can live a normal life without your gallbladder. Sometimes after the operation, you may have diarrhea if you eat foods that have too much fat, such as fried or greasy foods.

Pancreatitis (inflamed pancreas):

The pancreas is an organ that is in the middle/left upper part of the belly. Its job is to produce chemicals to help break down the food that you eat, especially fatty food. Sometimes the pancreas can become inflamed (irritated); we call this pancreatitis. We know it is inflamed because of symptoms like belly pain and vomiting, or from a blood test that confirms that you have pancreatitis. Many things can cause the pancreas to be inflamed, including alcohol, medicines, stones in your gallbladder, and germs. Pancreatitis pain can be treated with pain medicine. Pain medicine and hydration will be given intravenously while you fast, so that your gut can rest.

Small Bowel Obstruction (intestinal blockage):

The intestines are essentially very long pipes or tubes with multiple turns. Sometimes a piece of that pipe can have a kink, which means food will be unable to pass through smoothly. Symptoms such as stated, belly pain, bloating and constipation are indications of an intestinal blockage small bowel obstruction. The initial treatment may include placing a tube into your stomach through your mouth to decompress the intestines. An intestinal obstruction can require an operation if the tube option does not work.

Intestinal Bleeding:

Within the wall of the intestinal pipes are blood vessels. Sometimes the lining of the wall of the intestines gets damaged and those blood vessels start to leak. When this happens, bleeding inside the pipe makes its way down to your rectum. The bleeding can present in a variety of colors depending on the time the blood takes to travel through the intestines, and where in the intestines the bleeding started. For example, bleeding from the upper part of the pipe, like your stomach, will make your stool look black; while bleeding from the lower part of the pipe will make the stool look closer to actual blood (bright red).

Diverticulitis:

The intestines are made up of small and large pipes: small and large intestines. Sometimes, pockets develop in the wall of the large intestine (the large pipe that helps you absorb your food), and those pockets can get infected by bacteria. That infection is called diverticulitis. Usually medication (antibiotics) can take care of the infection and prevent the intestine from bursting. If the infection in the large intestine causes the wall of that pipe to burst, you may need an operation to have it fixed.

Appendicitis:

The appendix is a small organ that looks like a mini cucumber on the bottom right side of your belly. It serves no purpose that we know of. Sometimes bacteria from your intestines gets in there and causes it to be infected. Usually, an operation to remove it is required for the infection to be treated. You can live just fine without your appendix.

Hepatitis (liver inflammation/infection):

Your liver is located in the right upper part of your belly. Its job is to help you digest food and remove bad chemicals from your blood. Viruses, alcohol, and some medicines can cause your liver to get inflamed. That condition is called hepatitis.

Colitis:

Your gut is made up of small pipes (small intestines) and large pipes (large intestines). Both types of pipes can get inflamed. When the wall of the large intestine is inflamed, it's called colitis.

Perforated Bowel:

Your gut is like pipes that transport food through your body and get rid of the waste through your poop. Infection or injury can lead to holes in the wall of your gut. Food and fecal material that were supposed to be contained in those gut pipes are now floating inside the belly cavity. Fecal material has a lot of bacteria and so this situation can lead to a severe infection, if it is allowed to remain in your belly cavity.

Endocrine

Diabetes:

When you eat, your body turns food into sugars, or glucose. At that point, an organ in your belly, the pancreas, makes a substance called insulin. Insulin is the key that creates pathways for sugar to enter your muscles, tissues, and brain - so as to be used for energy. But with diabetes, this system does not work. Sometimes your body will make enough insulin, but the key doesn't work. This is called insulin resistance, and it is linked to Type 2 Diabetes. Type 2 Diabetes often happens when you are overweight. Diet and exercise, as well as oral medications are helpful to help reduce insulin resistance and get diabetes under control. Sometimes, after having Type 2 Diabetes for a long time, insulin injections are necessary. Type 1 Diabetes occurs when your immune system mistakenly attacks your pancreas and destroys the cells that make insulin. Without insulin, there is no mechanism that turns the sugar into energy for use by the cells, and so the cells starve because of lack of sugar, and the sugar builds up in the blood. The treatment for Type 1 Diabetes is insulin injections. The body can use this outside insulin to bring sugar into the body's cells. If left untreated, the high level of blood sugar from both types of Diabetes can damage your eyes, kidneys, nerves, heart, and can also lead to coma and to death.

Thyroid Disease:

The thyroid is a gland located in the front of your neck. It produces hormones that control every function in your body. When the thyroid does not work properly, it can present through a variety of symptoms. The symptoms will depend on the organ that is affected. Thyroid issues can be evaluated by blood tests. Most thyroid issues can be addressed by your primary care doctor.

Hyperglycemia:

The sugar level in your blood is above normal

D50, D10:

Please use term "Sugar water"

UROLOGICAL

Kidney Stones:

You have two organs at the sides of your lower back that produce urine (pee). These organs are called kidneys. The urine they produce is carried down to your bladder (a bag that holds urine) by a pipe called a ureter. Each kidney has its own ureter. Sometimes if you do not drink enough water, if your parents have a history of having stones in their kidneys, or if your pee has too many minerals, stones start to pile up in your kidney. Stones that are inside your kidney do not hurt. But when they leave the kidney and move through the very thin pipe called the ureter, they will cause intense pain until they make it to the bladder. There are a few ways to treat kidney stones. Usually, we give medicines for the pain, and to expand the ureter (the tube from your kidney to your bladder) to allow the stone to pass more easily.

Pyelonephritis (kidney infection):

You have two organs at the sides of your lower back called kidneys. They produce urine (pee). The urine is carried down to your bladder (bag that holds urine) by a pipe (ureter). An infection can start in your bladder and make its way up that pipe to your kidneys. The kidney infection is called pyelonephritis. Kidney infections usually have symptoms like flank pain, fever, nausea, vomiting, and symptoms of bladder infection like bloody /painful urine. Kidney infections can be treated at home with antibiotics tablets, or in the hospital intravenously, if the infection is severe and if you are unable to take antibiotics by mouth.

Urinary Retention:

The bladder is meant to hold a specific amount of urine. When the draining system of the bladder is blocked, the bladder retains more urine than it should. This causes discomfort of the lower belly along with decreased urine production. Urinary retention is treated by placing a tube through the penis or urethra to help temporarily relieve the obstruction and drain the bladder.

Urinary Tract Infection (bladder infection):

Your bladder is a balloon that holds your pee. A bladder infection occurs when a germ gets into the bladder. This can make you feel like you have to pee frequently, and it may cause pain or bleeding. Most often, bladder infections happen when germs from your gut (poop) get into the hole you pee from. You can avoid getting a bladder infection by peeing before and after you have sex, by wiping from front to back, and by peeing whenever you feel like you need to. A bladder infection can be treated with antibiotics.

Obstetrics

Ectopic Pregnancy:

Normally, when you are pregnant the baby grows in the uterus. Sometimes, the pregnancy can grow outside the uterus, in a tube between the uterus and the ovary or in the ovary. That is called an ectopic pregnancy. An ectopic pregnancy can be very dangerous if it ruptures. That can be treated by surgery or medication.

UROGENITAL

Urethritis:

The pipe that carries urine from the bladder (and semen in men) to the exterior of the body in both men and women is called the urethra. That pipe can get infected by germs acquired by engaging in unprotected sex. The infection can cause a discharge from the tip of your penis or from the vagina, making it burn when you pee. The infection can be treated with antibiotics.

Cervicitis:

The cervix is the bottom tip of the uterus (where the baby grows). The cervix can get infected by germs acquired by engaging in unprotected sex. The infection can cause an unusual discharge from your vagina. The infection can be treated with antibiotics.

MUSCULOSKELETAL

Achilles Tendon Rupture:

The Achilles tendon is located right above the heel of the foot. It helps in walking and pushing the foot down. When it is damaged, it causes pain and leads to difficulty in walking or pushing the foot down. Treatment for an Achilles tendon rupture will depend on the extent of the tear and the patient's activity status.

ACL Tear:

The ACL is a tendon in the knee that prevents the lower leg from extending too far. That tendon, when ruptured, leads to an unstable knee. Patients usually complain of knee buckling when attempting to walk on the involved leg. ACL treatment will depend on the extent of the tear and the patient's activity status.

Compression Fracture:

A compression fracture is a flattening of one of the blocks (vertebrae) that make up the spine. That flattening can be caused by a traumatic event such as a fall. The resulting symptoms will depend on the nearby structures affected by the pancaked vertebrae. Treatment will depend on the extent of the impact of the compression on surrounding vertebrae, as well as on your pain level.

Herniated Disc:

The spine is made of blocks of bones called vertebrae. In between those blocks there are discs which serve as shock absorbers for the spine. Once in a while, those discs can slip out of position. We call that a herniated disc. The slippage usually does not cause any symptoms unless the slipped disc pushes on a nerve. At this point, the slipped disc can cause symptoms ranging from pain to the inability to feel or move the impacted body part. Treatment will depend on the symptoms associated with the herniated disc.

Osteomyelitis (bone infection):

This is an infection in your bones. People who have diabetes, HIV, or those who shoot drugs in their veins are more likely to get this condition. The treatment for this kind of infection is antibiotics given intravenously.

Sciatica:

Sciatica is an inflammation of the sciatic nerve. The sciatic nerves originate from your lower spine and travel down the back of your legs to your feet. The nerves can get inflamed at any point along this path. That inflammation can come with burning pain that travels down the back of the leg(s), and more severe nerve issues if there is more substantial damage to the nerve(s). Sciatica is initially treated with anti-inflammatory muscle relaxants.

Strain:

When the tissue that connects muscles to bones stretches too far, it's called a strain. Treatment includes rest, ice, and elevation of the involved extremity.

Sprain:

When the tissue that connects two bones stretches too far, it's called a sprain. Treatment includes rest, ice, elevation of involved extremity.

Skin

Cellulitis:

Cellulitis is a skin infection. Sometimes bacteria that is supposed to be outside the skin gets underneath the skin and starts to multiply, causing the redness and warmth that comes with this infection. That illness occurs more often in people whose body cannot fight off the bacteria, like those with diabetes or cancer. Cellulitis is treated by taking medications called antibiotics.

Abscess:

An abscess is an infection underneath the skin. It presents as a painful bump on the skin. The bump may have a hole with pus coming out of it, some redness over the infection, and may be warmer than other parts of the body. The bump can also feel squishy. People who have diabetes are more likely to get abscesses. An abscess can be treated by numbing the area and draining the pus out. Antibiotics taken orally can be used as well.

Shingles:

Shingles is a skin infection that is caused by a virus. It's the same virus that causes chickenpox. After you've had chickenpox, the virus lives in the nerves of your spine and can come back years later as shingles. The rash is usually painful and follows a specific pattern that matches the path of the infected nerve. The rash is contagious while it is open and releasing pus. Treatment includes antiviral medicines, steroids (strong anti-inflammation medication), and pain medications.

Oncological

Cancer:

Cancer is a condition where some cells in your body are not behaving the way they were intended to. In some cases, those cells can lead to the creation of a mass. In other cases, we need more specific tests to find those abnormal cells.

Leukemia:

There are trillions of cells in the body, including blood cells. White blood cells help fight infections in the body. Those white blood cells can start to replicate abnormally fast and create cells that do not function well. That process is called leukemia. The treatment of leukemia depends on a number of factors that can be explained by a cancer specialist (oncologist).

Lymphoma:

The immune system is made up of a variety of tissues scattered throughout the body. Lymphocytes are types of cells that help to fight infections. If these cells grow out of control, the result can be changes in their structure. That process is called Lymphoma. The treatment of lymphoma depends on a number of factors that can be explained by a cancer specialist (oncologist).

Hematological

Anemia:

Blood is the transporter of nutrients to all parts of the body. It maintains a certain amount of iron and hemoglobin in your system. Normal levels of hemoglobin from a blood test should be between 12 and 14 (depending on the lab). If your number falls below that range, you are considered to be anemic. There are a number of conditions that can cause anemia, and the treatment is dependent on the underlying condition.

Infectious Disease

Bacteria vs Viruses:

Bacteria and Viruses are both organisms we cannot see with our eyes, but they can cause all kinds of infections such as colds, bronchitis, pneumonia and even COVID-19. The important thing to know about them is that antibiotics do not kill viruses. Antibiotics only work on bacteria.

Sepsis, bacteremia (Blood infection):

Bacteria that cause infections in organs like the lungs or bladder, can leave those organs and get into your bloodstream. If they get into your blood they can cause a general infection in your body leading to symptoms like fever or marked blood pressure drop, which will make you feel weak and dizzy. Treatment for sepsis is antibiotics taken through an (IV) directly in your vein.

Q Quiz: Patient Speak

98. Washing of hands before touching anyone or anything is the best way to prevent the spread of conjunctivitis.

    A. True

    B. False

    Answer: A

99. Which of the following is the medical terminology for when the blood flow to the brain is blocked?"

    A. Aortic Aneurysm

    B. Heart Attack

    C. Stroke

    D. Pleural Effusion

    Answer: C

100. A family member has brought in a patient and is sure that they have had a stroke. It is important to explain to the family member that the patient may have _____, since the symptoms are the same as a stroke.

    A. Low blood sugar

    B. Hypertension

    C. Pulmonary Embolism

    D. Pancreatitis

    Answer: A

101. When initiating the involuntary institutionalization, you must inform the patient and family that the length of detainment will be maximum of:

A. 24 hours

B. 48 hours

C. 72 hours

D. 72 hours or when cleared by a licensed psychiatrist

Answer: D

102. You can verify a suspected heart attack by: :

A. EKG results

B. Detecting a chemical released by the heart muscle when it is not getting enough blood flow called troponin

C. Testing for blood-borne pathogens

D. Answers A and B above

Answer: D

103. Which of the following is best explained to a patient by saying the following: "The heart sits in a sac. The sac can fill with fluid, which might be associated with an infection or from cancer. There is a surgical procedure to remove that fluid."

A. Colitis

B. Myocardial Infarction

C. Pericardial Effusion

D. Pneumonia

Answer: C

104. Which of the following layman's descriptions will best explain the cause of asthma to a patient?

    A. A condition that causes the lining of the lungs to be irritated and swollen.

    B. An infection of the lungs caused by a bacteria, fungus, or virus.

    C. Air escaping the lungs and entering the chest cavity.

    D. A blood clot in an artery within the lungs.

    Answer: A

105. Which layman's description will best explain the cause of pneumonia?

    A. A condition that causes the lining of the lungs to be irritated and swollen.

    B. An infection of the lungs caused by a bacteria, fungus, or virus.

    C. Fluid entering the space between the lungs and a cover of tissue.

    D. Air escaping the lungs and entering the chest cavity.

    Answer: B

106. If a heavy nicotine smoker tells you that smoking can't cause a stomach ulcer because the stomach is not in the lungs, you will need to explain to them that smoking nicotine can cause a stomach ulcer and several other intestinal and non-intestinal conditions.

    A. True

    B. False

    Answer: A

107. A patient has extreme anxiety over the idea of having any type of surgery because their father passed during a routine procedure. If the patient has gallstones, you need to inform them that their options are?

   A. Changing their diet i.e., adopting a fat free diet.

   B. Starting a protocol of medication.

   C. Having an operation to remove the gallbladder.

   D. Answers A and C only.

   Answer: D

108. Which layman's description will best explain diverticulitis to your patient?

   A. A blood vessel that is leaking blood into the colon from a damaged lining.

   B. A bacterial infection of the lining of the pocket(s) of your large intestine, typically caused by persistent constipation.

   C. Inflammation of the pancreas causes vomiting.

   D. Irritation of the stomach lining caused by certain foods or smoking.

   Answer: B

109. Patients can live without any dietary adjustments when this organ is removed.

   A. Appendix

   B. Gallbladder

C. Pancreas

D. Liver

Answer: A

110. Which organ may best be described to a patient by saying that it filters the blood of bad chemicals, helps digest food, and when inflamed, causes a condition we call hepatitis?

A. Colon

B. Gallbladder

C. Liver

D. Small intestine

Answer: C

111. If an older patient is overweight, is sedentary, and is eating poorly, you need to discuss the risk of type II diabetes and advise them to change their lifestyle.

A. True

B. False

Answer: A

112. True or False? A layman's description of hyperglycemia is that the sugar level in the blood is below normal.

A. True

B. False

Answer: B

113. When discussing kidney stones with a patient, explain that the pain from the stones occurs when the stone:

    A. Is in the kidney.

    B. Is in the bladder.

    C. Is moving through the ureter (pipe that connects kidney to bladder).

    D. Is moving through the urethra.

    Answer: C

114. To prevent urinary tract infections, you should inform patients to:

    A. Urinate both prior to and after sex

    B. Wipe from front to back

    C. Urinate when they need and not hold it

    D. All the above recommendations

    Answer: D

115. A female patient has cervicitis and has admitted that they engage in high-risk sexual activities with more than one partner. You need to inform them that using condoms can help prevent cervicitis and some other STDs in the future if they choose not to change their lifestyle.

    A. True

    B. False

    Answer: A

116. True or False? When explaining to a patient the difference between a strain and a sprain, it would be accurate to depict a strain as affecting the tissues connecting bone to bone.

   A. True

   B. False

   Answer: B

117. Which of the following is best explained to a patient by stating the following: "White blood cells help fight infections in the body, but sometimes they start to replicate abnormally fast and create cells that do not function well."

   A. Anemia

   B. Osteomyelitis

   C. Leukemia

   D. Sepsis

   Answer: C

118. True or False? During trauma assessments it is important to explain to the patient everything that is happening to them and around them during the exam.

   A. True

   B. False

   Answer: A

119. When prescribing a medication, you should explain why the medication is needed, what the medication will do, what the possible side effects may be, and the future desired state after taking the medication.

    A. True

    B. False

    Answer: A

120. It is important to explain the risk of radiation exposure to a patient prior to sending them for a:

    A. CT scan or MRI

    B. MRI or Ultrasound

    C. CT Scan or X-Ray

    D. Ultrasound or X-Ray

    Answer: C

121. When assessing internal injuries or conditions, it may be important to explain the role of PO contrasts to a patient, and tell them to expect the entire process to last about:

    A. 1 hour

    B. 2 hours

    C. Always overestimate the time particular studies may take as many factors impact the ultimate completion of that study. Furthermore, if the study is performed in a shorter timeframe the patient is pleasantly surprised and the provider is their new hero.

    D. 4 hours

    Answer: C

122. Regarding incidental findings during imaging, it can be best practice to:

    A. Print out a copy of the image or report for the patient /Refer the patient to the patient portal

    B. Let the patient know the incidental image is not related to your diagnosis.

    C. Inform the patient to follow up with their PCP as soon as possible.

    D. All the above are best practices.

    Answer: D

123. True or False? When explaining a Foley Catheter, you could say that a Foley Catheter is a tube that will be placed in the patient's bladder through the penis/ure-thra to drain urine and to monitor urine output.

    A. True

    B. False

    Answer: A

SECTION FIVE

CASE STUDIES

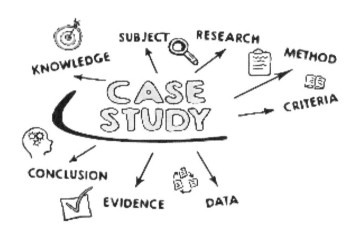

CASE 1

A 46 year old female in bed 52 is demanding the covid 19 monoclonal antibody. She has no underlying medical history. She has a Ph.D. and introduces herself as "doctor." She is having mild symptoms. Her physician is my colleague and has made it abundantly clear to her that she does not qualify for that treatment. She disagrees. After multiple failed attempts to achieve accord, my colleague asks me to intervene.

I review the chart, the lab results and x-ray findings. All completely unremarkable. I make my way to see the patient. I knock and enter the room. She is seated on the bed and appears comfortable. I introduce myself, my role in the ER and I say, "I am sorry for the inconvenience." Then I ask, "How can we help you?" As she starts to explain her issue I take a seat a couple feet from her. She details her symptoms as well as her concerns. She makes constant reference to the fact that she had called our ER to find out if she would be able to get the monoclonal treatment, and that she had been assured that she would get it by a non-medical staff member.

After she presents her concerns to me I apologize again for her ordeal and explain that the person she spoke to should not have given her that assurance. I apologize once again for our error and tell her that our nursing director will instruct all our secretarial staff to refrain from giving medical advice over the phone. I then review her vital signs, blood work and x-rays, reconfirming that she does not in fact need the treatment she was asking for. I give her the opportunity to ask questions, but she declines. Lastly, I give her my business card and detail the specific symptoms that would demand either a call to me or a visit to the emergency room.

After I left this patient's room, I never heard from her. I never got a complaint. I asked our nursing leadership team to address the issue with the staff.

Lessons Learned:

Apology

Starting with a heartfelt apology in what might be a confrontational situation disarms the aggrieved party. It sets the tone for the whole interaction. I encourage you to apologize to any disgruntled patient who comes your way, whether you are at fault or not.

Sitting Down

Sitting down puts you at or below eye level of the other party. It is a non-confrontational position. It tells the patient that you are here for as long as it takes and that you are interested in finding a solution to their problem.

Listening

Truly listening, encouraging the patient to vent is how I was able to understand her real issue: she felt that she had been lied to. The patient clearly felt that the lie (she would get monoclonal antibodies) required an apology and a mechanism to make sure that similar situations would not occur moving forward.

Process error

We had a flawed process. The secretarial staff should not have given medical advice to anyone unless it had been cleared with a physician. This patient's persistence allowed us to discover that kink in our process. We were lucky that we did not have a bad outcome from that issue. Patient complaints can help prevent poor outcomes and identify flaws in our process, if we take the time to listen, to analyze the situation, and to place it in the broader context of patient care.

CASE 2

A 90-year-old gentleman comes in complaining of a mechanical (trip) fall. The patient drove himself to the hospital. He recalls every aspect of the fall. He complains of an abrasion at the top of his scalp and denies any other symptoms. He is not on a blood thinner. The exam elicits some minimal pain at the center of his upper neck around C2. The patient is placed in a C-Collar. An initial work up is initiated that includes a CT of his brain and cervical spine. As we wait for the results of the CTs, the patient's wife shows up. She confirms that he fell and adds that she had found him on the floor. When she found him he told her that he had fallen six hours prior and had remained on the floor. The new piece of information provided by his wife prompts us to conduct further blood tests which result in a diagnosis of rhabdomyolysis and acute kidney injury in addition to his neck fractures.

Lesson:

Patients may willfully or accidentally omit key information that could be helpful in their management. As medical detectives, we must be open to collecting as much information as possible to help us optimally manage our patients. We have to create an environment within which the patient's loved ones feel comfortable about participating in their care.

CASE 3

A 28-year-old male comes in complaining of upper abdominal pain after eating at a Subway restaurant two hours prior. He has three episodes of non-bloody/non-bilious vomiting. The work up is completely negative. The patient is hydrated and receives some medication for his nausea and abdominal pain. He says he feels 100 percent better and is discharged home. A day later,

I get a call from the patient stating that his abdominal pain has returned. The pain is now located in the right lower abdomen. Additionally, the patient does not feel like eating and has subjective fevers. I ask him to promptly return to the ER to see me. On the reevaluation he is now tender at the right lower abdominal quadrant and guarding. The CT of his belly confirms appendicitis. He has an appendectomy and an uneventful recovery.

Lesson:

Patient care is not limited to the walls of our healthcare centers. A patient leaving our offices must still be able to easily resolve issues that arise. I was more than happy to have that patient call back with new symptoms, and happy that I was able to help. The patient had a great outcome and there were no legal consequences.

CASE 4

"The patient in hallway N keeps sweating" says the nurse just as I am about to see another patient. I look at her, intrigued. She adds "Yeah, it looks like he has been running a marathon except he has been laying in his gurney for the last 20 minutes." I promptly followed the nurse to the patient's location. On my initial exam the patient is profusely diaphoretic. On further questioning, the patient simply complains of "not feeling right." The only pertinent history: the patient has a longstanding history of tobacco use.

After the physical exam, I rush back to my desk and call the CT department to ask them to immediately scan the patient's chest, abdomen, and pelvis. As soon as the scan is done, I get a call from the CT asking me to immediately look at the study.

Within minutes the patient is sent to our main sister hospital. The patient survives his aortic dissection.

If it were not for the prompt thinking of this nurse, the patient would have had a poor outcome. Creating an environment where the ancillary staff feels valued and where their input/ questions are welcomed maximizes the potential for a positive patient outcome. The ancillary staff are our eyes and ears while the patients are under our care. Every member of my staff is a model for the "best practices" of their profession while interacting with patients. In response to my 'boasts' about them, and to the open communication work environment, they work very hard to meet my expectations of them, and they are able to bring their valuable medical experience to bear when they share their thoughts and opinions about our patients.

CASE 6

This case is about a patient who disagrees with their provider. Mrs. Jones is in room 10. Before walking in, the nurse gives me a heads up - "You are going to need some time!" Very early on during the medical interview, Mrs. Jones makes it clear that she doesn't believe in medications or vaccines. She thinks that "drug companies" are only trying to make money from "suckers." During the visit, I try to answer her questions by referring to medical data and uncomplicated terminology. At the end of the visit, the patient remains unmoved: she will not take any medications or vaccines.

It is completely acceptable for a patient to reject the evidence-based advice brought forward by a provider. We are teachers/

advisers. Any of our patients can refuse our advice. Our job is to ensure that we are giving them evidence-based advice and that it is understood. Be respectful of anyone who disagrees with your medical recommendations. Do not get offended.

CASE 7

A 24-year-old female calls her gynecologist's office to schedule an appointment for her yearly exam. She has a poor experience with the front desk. Upon reviewing the patient's records, the office staff notice that the patient has missed the previous two appointments. The staff member abruptly starts to berate the patient about missing the appointments and tells the patient that she should not "waste our time." As the office staff member goes on, the patient is reminded of the painful reasons that had forced her to miss her appointments. Distraught, the patient politely hangs up and goes online to look for a new gynecologist.

Lesson:

The patient experience must involve everyone and begins the moment the patient decides to visit your healthcare center. Your job is to ensure that they can navigate the different stations of their visit successfully and with empathy. For that to happen, everyone involved directly or indirectly in the care of the patient must be on the same page. Everyone must understand their role and must be trained to the point that they can deliver a great patient experience and be held accountable if they fail to do so.

CASE 8

A 95-year-old male in bed 4 is complaining of generalized weakness. He tells the resident that he used to be a producer of an international fashion show and is usually very healthy. He asks the resident about their background, family etc. He tells the resident that he likes the food at this hospital better than the other hospitals, which is why he told the ambulance to bring him here. The resident becomes visibly frustrated with all the talking the patient is doing and repeatedly interrupts him to try to "take a good history." Eventually, the patient stops talking. The resident tells the attending staff that the patient is fine and just came to the hospital for food. A few days later the patient ends up in the ER in acute CHF.

Lesson:

Don't be quick to interrupt a patient. Patients do not know that physicians are programmed to look for specific clues when they talk. Those clues help our trained brains to create differential diagnoses. It is common for patients to talk about topics that are "irrelevant" during the medical interview. Those personal tidbits being shared help build rapport and give us a window into the patient's life. Remember, when a patient shares details about their lives, they are testing us to see if we are really listening so that they know they can trust us. If they do not feel comfortable, they will not trust. If they don't trust you, they won't follow your treatment plan. Listen to your patients. The information they share will help us formulate medical and social plans to maximize our patient's outcome. It is always important to remember that social determinants of health can impact patient outcomes. The patient in this case study is likely suffering from social isolation and food insecurity. Paying close attention to what patients are saying can lead clinicians to involve social workers or other care teams. In this case, a listening resident could have prevented a poor outcome for the patient.

CASE 9

A 31 year-old male is found unconscious at home by rescue. He is given Narcan and wakes up. Upon reaching the facility, the patient is fully awake and refuses any blood work: "I don't do any drugs. "I play basketball" is the answer he provides every time he is asked about using opiates. Eventually the patient leaves the facility against medical advice, and under the care of his brother. Three hours later a physician from a neighboring facility. calls in to report that he is seeing the patient who left against medical advice. He reports that the patient ended up at his facility in respiratory distress and was placed on a ventilator. The secondary physician reports some of the findings: WBC: 31, Lactic acid of 7.

Lesson:

Biases can quickly turn a patient off and potentially lead to poor outcomes. Once that bias is perceived, patients will be hesitant about sharing any information that may help in their workup. When patients are approached with biases, they tend to recoil and shy away from our prescriptive advice. These patients are wary of our medical advice because they wonder what biases are informing it.

CASE 10

You recently find out that one of your colleagues has committed suicide. Apparently, your colleague found out five years before that his wife had been cheating on him throughout their 20 years of marriage. He went through a painful divorce and lost most of his retirement savings because of it. He then lost his house and the family dog. Throughout his tenure at your center this colleague had exemplary clinical conduct and was loved by the staff. Overall, he seemed content with his life

Appearances can be deceiving. Some people are naturally very forthcoming with their personal challenges; most of us in healthcare are not. Most of us believe that we are not supposed to have everyday challenges and if we somehow do have them, we must not talk about them. Because we see so many horrors in healthcare practice, we have trained ourselves to shut down our emotions so that we can function while dealing with patient emergencies. Unfortunately, medical training programs some-times teach us to be "less" human and do little to prepare us to support each other or be supported while we are on the job. It is important to remember that challenges are part of the human condition, and that providers are human and not divine. We sur-vive by checking in on each other. Not the perfunctory kind of checking in but the kind that tells the other person that you see them, that you care about them, and that you are there to sup-port them if needed.

CASE 11

A patient narrates her experience in the ER. "I went to the emer-gency room with a heavy feeling in my chest and was concerned about fainting. I am asthmatic and I know when I'm having an asthma attack, and this was not it. I also suffer from panic attacks, and this was also not it. I've never fainted before. The only things they did were to order some general blood/lab work and a chest X-ray. What about my fainting? A cat scan or Head CT should've been completed, but it wasn't called for. I felt that the doctors weren't really listening to me, and just wanted to clear up the bed in the hallway to bring in another patient."

Lesson:

Take the time to explain to patients WHY you are only ordering the tests you have asked for, discuss the results with them, and explain why the tests done are enough. Use language that is non-technical, and that the patient will in turn be able to use when explaining their condition to family members or friends who are not in the medical field.

CONCLUSION

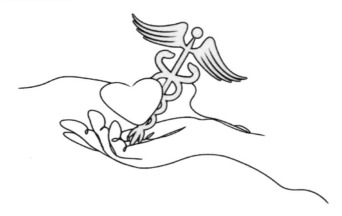

I am often asked how I continue to be excited about patient care and emergency medicine after all those years, "especially in light of"…(fill with whatever negative trope you can imagine)? There are multiple reasons I am passionate about coming to work every day. I believe it's what I was meant to do.

At one point in my life, I wanted to pursue a Ph.D. in immunology and worked at the National Institute of Health (NIH). I quickly realized that bench work—away from patients—did not fit my personality and was not satisfying to me. Clinical work and patient interaction were my superpower years later, I remain excited about interacting with patients and helping their medical conditions. It is truly gratifying to help others on their journey to physical and mental health. I encourage everyone working in healthcare—particularly with the challenges we face daily— to remind ourselves of the extraordinary and positive impact we can have on others. As a lifelong medical practitioner, I am always looking for ways to improve our commitment to our patients and to provide the best care possible for them. It was during my MBA class that the idea of team building often done in Corporate America sparked an idea for team building and my development of procedures for team building in my own institution. Being open, forward thinking, and current can be a benefit to all. The worst thing anyone can ever say is, "We have always done it that way." I encourage you to be innovative, open minded and compassionate.

Here are the reasons why I remain passionate about my chosen profession:

Perspective : I was lucky to be born in Haiti, an amazing country with multiple challenges. I lived there for the first 18 years of my life and have returned home frequently over the years. Growing up in Haiti instilled in me an appreciation for medical care, which is not as prevalent there as it is in the U.S. Each interaction with a medical professional in Haiti is cherished by the lucky few who receive it. I carry that sentiment with me to this day.

Leadership: Hillel says, "If I am not for myself, who will be for me? If I am only for myself, what am I? And if not now, when?" Leadership matters, and I often ask myself, "If I don't do it, how can I expect others to?" I absolutely believe that the positive patient experience starts with effective leadership at medical facilities. Medical and non-medical personnel who "walk the walk," set the tone, and create the behavioral template for others to follow.

Colleagues. It is easy to enjoy your job if you appreciate those with whom you work, and if they appreciate you too. If your team understands that everything you do is centered around your patient's welfare, they will respect you and emulate your behavior.

Balance : Medicine, as with everything else in life, requires balance. Healthcare is physically, intellectually, emotionally, and psychologically draining. Every healthcare provider must have an outlet that allows them to reset both physically and emotionally. To achieve that balance, the provider must conduct frequent self-assessments to determine when a break is needed. In my case, when I am not working clinically I spend time with my family. I love being with my family. I also do a lot of exercising (running) and gardening. Then too, my wife and I started a nonprofit—Primary Care Haiti—a few years ago. We take tremendous joy in training healthcare providers in Haiti so that they in turn can train others to carry out interventions like cardiac resuscitation, ACLS, BLS, ultrasound. These are things that I enjoy doing, and so they are the outlets that give me the breaks that I need to balance my life.

Empathy. When we're not at our best, we may think of our patients as "stubborn" or "non-compliant." It might be wiser to look in the mirror and realize that a that moment our listening and communications skills are lacking. I constantly remind myself to try to understand where my patients are coming from and to give them the benefit of the doubt. An empathetic approach will likely lead to trust, the most important ingredient in any successful patient-provider relationship. From trust comes the pathways we can use to help the patients on the road to recovery. And isn't that why we chose to be providers of care in the first place?

ACKNOWLEDGEMENTS

There are a number of people who have contributed to the completion of this manual.

My father-in-law, Steven Rakitt. Thank you for being my de facto initial editor of this manuscript. Thank you for your willingness to look at every page I sent you and for your skill in distilling my words to their most impactful meaning.

My ER residents, Dr. Sarah Eldin and Dr. Matthew Bidwell. Thank you for sharing your perspective as trainees and adding some relevant commentary to this Manual.

My sister, Sarah Telson, JD, for the Gender and Identity section.

Gloria Almodovar (ER Nurse Director), LaShonda Rogers (Unit Coordinator), Michael Rodriguez (Medic, Firefighter), Deedra Satahoo (ER Nurse). Thank you for taking the time to share your insights.

Medical student, Dr. Jonathan Munoz. Thank you for sharing your perspective as a medical student. Thank you for being a great scribe and eagerly participating in our training program in Haiti.

To my mother-in-law, Sandy Mahoney, thank you for your eternal support.

To my siblings. I love you.

To my boys. Thank you for being who you are. Never be afraid to put your core beliefs on display as long as you believe in your deepest core that you are doing the right thing and it makes you happy.

To my wife, Dr Jennifer Goldman. You are my rock. Thank you for encouraging me for the past six plus years to put this manuscript together. Thank you for seeing the need for this. Thank you for believing that my voice would resonate with those in need of such training. Thank you for your objectivity, your support, and your unconditional love.

A supplement to the print and eBook versions of this guide is our online training system: www.howtopatient.com.

How To Patient: *howtopatient.com* is a training website that is a supplement to the print and eBook versions of *Doctor Goldman's Guide to Effective Patient Communication Explanations of the Most Common Medical Conditions in Layperson's Terms and Helpful Provider-Patient Interactions*

How To Patient is a self-improvement tool. It fosters continuing learning and encourages users to accept that they may not always have the perfect approach when dealing with patients. How To Patient enhances the current medical education curriculum and provides training in communication and patient care. www.howtopatient.com was created to fill in the gaps and provide much-needed guidance in these areas.

Made in the USA
Monee, IL
14 September 2023